BestMasters

Springer awards „BestMasters" to the best master's theses which have been completed at renowned universities in Germany, Austria, and Switzerland.

The studies received highest marks and were recommended for publication by supervisors. They address current issues from various fields of research in natural sciences, psychology, technology, and economics.

The series addresses practitioners as well as scientists and, in particular, offers guidance for early stage researchers.

Hanna Birke

Model-Based Recursive Partitioning with Adjustment for Measurement Error

Applied to the Cox's Proportional Hazards and Weibull Model

Foreword by Prof. Dr. Thomas Augustin

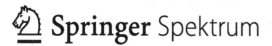 **Springer** Spektrum

Hanna Birke
Düsseldorf, Germany

BestMasters
ISBN 978-3-658-08504-9   ISBN 978-3-658-08505-6 (eBook)
DOI 10.1007/978-3-658-08505-6

Library of Congress Control Number: 2015930262

Springer Spektrum
© Springer Fachmedien Wiesbaden 2015

Printed on acid-free paper

Springer Spektrum is a brand of Springer Fachmedien Wiesbaden
Springer Fachmedien Wiesbaden is part of Springer Science+Business Media
(www.springer.com)

Foreword

In recent years data-analytic methods originating from the area of machine learning have gained also strong momentum in Statistics. Statisticians have contributed to the methodological foundations of these algorithmic methods and substantially extended them, and thus these methods have become part of statistical methodology. A particularly popular example are recursive partitioning methods, including so-called classification and regression trees. Their basic rationale is to analyse multivariate data by successively splitting the sample and thus partitioning it into sub-groups that are homogeneous with respect to an outcome variable of interest. Originally, these methods, which are typically very powerful in prediction problems, have been understood as model-free, providing a fundamental alternative to regression modelling, contrasting the explanation-oriented regression modelling culture with the prediction-oriented algorithmic culture.

This seemingly fundamental antagonism is overcome by the model-based recursive partitioning ("MOB") approach of Zeileis, Hothorn & Hornik (2008; Journal of Computational and Graphical Statistics), where, in simplified terms, regression models are spilt: First a regression model relating the core covariates to the response variable is estimated on the whole sample, and then it is investigated for parameter instability, i.e. whether the individual score contributions suggest a substantial structural change in the parameter values over the ordered values of some additional variable. If so, the sample is split, and separate regression models are estimated for the sub-groups, which then are taken as new samples for an iterative repetition of the procedures until a stopping criterion is fulfilled. In the end, the procedure gives the user a partition whose members are homogeneous with respect to the core regression model, and thus parsimonious regression models of high explanatory power are obtained - if (!) no measurement error occurs.

However, substantial measurement error is quite a common problem, for instance, in econometrics and biometrics. Therefore, the development of powerful measurement correction methods has been an intensively studied area in traditional regression models. Birke is the first who transferred some of these methods to the model-based recursive partitioning context. Her basic technical insight is that for the MOB methodology it is sufficient to consider arbitrary unbiased estimation functions, instead of the commonly used likelihood-based score-function. Birke therefore relies on measurement error corrected score functions in terms of Nakamura, and she is indeed able to extend the whole MOB framework to the situation of classical additive covariate measurement error. This includes a sophisticated implementation for the Weibull and the Cox model that makes this computationally quite demanding procedure still practically applicable. A well designed simulation study corroborates the high power of the developed methodology.

By incorporating measurement error correction methods in a very elegant and efficient way, Birke's work boosts the practical application and relevance of the model-based recursive partitioning methodology.

Munich, November 2014   *Prof. Dr. Thomas Augustin*

Short Profile of the Working Group

The working group *Foundations of Statistics and Their Applications* (head: Prof. Dr. Thomas Augustin; `www.statistik.lmu.de/institut/ag/agmg/index.html`) is one of eight working groups/chairs at the Department of Statistics at LMU Munich.

The research vision of the group is to contribute to the development of a powerful comprehensive statistical methodology where the often limited data quality is explicitly reflected in statistical modelling and inference. In contrast to traditional methods, which indispensably require strong, often empirically not tenable assumptions on data formation, the novel methods deliberately aim at drawing reliable conclusions from complex data, leading to deeper insights into social, economic and biological structures and processes.

Therefore one main focus of research is on reliable inference by set-valued methods (imprecise probabilities, partial identification) and (generalized) measurement error modelling. Further research interests include other issues in the foundations of statistical inference, statistical aspects of empirical social research and psychometrics, survival analysis, graphical models and different machine learning methods.

Acknowledgment

This master's thesis was written under the direction of Prof. Dr. Thomas Augustin at the Department of Statistics of the Ludwig-Maximilians-University Munich.

In particular, I would like to express my gratitude to Prof. Dr. Thomas Augustin for the interesting and relevant topic of the thesis, for the good cooperation as well as for his helpful and valuable suggestions. I appreciate his support at any time. In addition, I wish to thank Teresa for proofreading my thesis and for her constructive comments.

I would like to thank my 'stät girls' Ina, Kathrin, Sonja and Teresa as well as Markus. I am grateful to have found such amazing friends who have accompanied me throughout my studies.

Furthermore, I thank Jan, Michael, my sister Lena and especially my parents for their constant support and encouragement.

Düsseldorf, November 2014   *Hanna Birke*

Contents

1. Introduction 1

2. Theoretical Background 3
 2.1. Cox Model and Measurement Error 3
  2.1.1. Measurement Error Model 5
  2.1.2. Adjustment for Measurement Error in Cox Model 6
  2.1.3. Corrected Log-Likelihood and Score Function in Cox and
   Weibull Model 9
 2.2. Model-Based Recursive Partitioning 21
  2.2.1. Introduction to Classification and Regression Trees 22
  2.2.2. Model-Based Recursive Partitioning 24

3. Implementation 35
 3.1. Model-Based Recursive Partitioning in R 35
 3.2. Fitting a MOB Weibull Model with Adjustment for Measurement
  Error 39

4. Simulation Study 55
 4.1. Check the fit Function 56
  4.1.1. Check the fit Function - only W 57
  4.1.2. Check the fit Function - W and F 66
 4.2. Structural Changes 71
  4.2.1. Structural Changes - single 72
  4.2.2. Structural Changes - multi 80
 4.3. One Global Model Fit vs. MOB 85
 4.4. Conclusion of the Simulation Study 92

5. Conclusion 95

Appendix 101

A. R-Code   **101**

   A.1. *SurvRegcorr.r* 101

B. Proofs and Derivations   **107**

   B.1. Cox Model - Corrected Log-Likelihood 107

   B.2. Cox Model - Corrected Score Functions 108

   B.3. Weibull Model - Log-Likelihood 110

      B.3.1. Version 2 110

      B.3.2. Version 2 = Version 1 110

   B.4. Weibull Model - Corrected Log-Likelihood 111

   B.5. Weibull Model - Corrected Score Functions 113

   B.6. Weibull Model - Corrected Log-Likelihood with Interaction Term . 114

   B.7. Generating Failure Times 118

   B.8. Mean Expected Failure Time 119

C. Results of the Simulation Study   **121**

   C.1. Check the `fit` function - only W 121

      C.1.1. `beta.true` = -0.2, `tau.true` = -0.3, `prob.cens` = 35% and $V \sim N(0,1)$ 121

      C.1.2. `beta.true` = -0.2, `tau.true` = -0.3, `prob.cens` = 35% and $V \sim Unif(0,\sqrt{12})$ 131

      C.1.3. `beta.true` = 0.4, `tau.true` = 0.5, `prob.cens` = 0% and $V \sim N(0,1)$ 140

      C.1.4. `beta.true` = 0.4, `tau.true` = 0.5, `prob.cens` = 0% and $V \sim Unif(0,\sqrt{12})$ 149

   C.2. Check the `fit` function - W and F 158

      C.2.1. `beta.V.true` = 0.6, `beta.F.true` = -0.1, `tau.true` = -0.5, `prob.cens` = 0% and $V \sim N(0,1)$ 158

      C.2.2. `beta.V.true` = 0.6, `beta.F.true` = -0.1 , `tau.true` = -0.5, `prob.cens` = 0% and $V \sim Unif(0,\sqrt{12})$ 173

   C.3. Structural Changes - single 188

      C.3.1. `beta.1.true` = 0.6, `beta.2.true` = -0.2 , `tau.1.true` = 0.5, `tau.2.true` = -0.4, `prob.cens` = 35% and $V \sim N(0,1)$ 188

   C.4. Structural Changes - multi 209

      C.4.1. Summary of Parameter Estimation 218

C.5. One Global Model Fit vs. MOB 224

    C.5.1. `beta.1.true` $= 0.6$, `beta.2.true` $=$ -0.2 , `tau.1.true` $=$ 0.5, `tau.2.true` $=$ -0.4, `prob.cens` $= 0\%$ and $V \sim N(0,1)$. 224

Bibliography **235**

List of Figures

2.1. Recursive partitioning with Lung Cancer Data, generated in R with the function `ctree()` 23

2.2. MOB with Pima Indians data, generated in R with the function `mob()` 26

3.1. Model-based recursive partitioning with Lung Cancer Data 47

4.1. MOB estimated via the corrected approach with `beta.1.true` = 0.6, `beta.2.true` = -0.2 , `tau.1.true` = 0.5, `tau.2.true` = -0.4, `prob.cens` = 35%, $V \sim N(0,1)$, `size` = 1000 and `sd.U` = 0.4 . . . 74

4.2. MOB fitted via the corrected estimation with `beta.1.true` = -0.9, `beta.2.true` = 0.2 , `beta.3.true` = 1.1, `tau.1.true` = -1, `tau.2.true` = 0.1, `tau.3.true` = 0.9, `prob.cens` = 0%, $V \sim N(0,1)$, `size` = 1000 and `sd.U` = 0.4 81

C.1. Boxplot for β_V with `beta.true` = -0.2, `tau.true` = -0.3, `prob.cens` = 35%, $V \sim N(0,1)$, `size` = 100 122

C.2. Boxplot for τ with `beta.true` = -0.2, `tau.true` = -0.3, `prob.cens` = 35%, $V \sim N(0,1)$, `size` = 100 123

C.3. Boxplot for β_V with `beta.true` = -0.2, `tau.true` = -0.3, `prob.cens` = 35%, $V \sim N(0,1)$, `size` = 500 125

C.4. Boxplot for τ with `beta.true` = -0.2, `tau.true` = -0.3, `prob.cens` = 35%, $V \sim N(0,1)$, `size` = 500 126

C.5. Boxplot for β_V with `beta.true` = -0.2, `tau.true` = -0.3, `prob.cens` = 35%, $V \sim N(0,1)$, `size` = 1000 128

C.6. Boxplot for τ with `beta.true` = -0.2, `tau.true` = -0.3, `prob.cens` = 35%, $V \sim N(0,1)$, `size` = 1000 129

C.7. Boxplot for β_V with `beta.true` = -0.2, `tau.true` = -0.3, `prob.cens` = 35%, $V \sim Unif(0, \sqrt{12})$, `size` = 100 131

C.8. Boxplot for τ with `beta.true` = -0.2, `tau.true` = -0.3, `prob.cens` = 35%, $V \sim Unif(0, \sqrt{12})$, `size` = 100 132

C.9. Boxplot for β_V with beta.true = -0.2, tau.true = -0.3, prob.cens = 35%, $V \sim Unif(0, \sqrt{12})$, size = 500 134

C.10.Boxplot for τ with beta.true = -0.2, tau.true = -0.3, prob.cens = 35%, $V \sim Unif(0, \sqrt{12})$, size = 500 135

C.11.Boxplot for β_V with beta.true = -0.2, tau.true = -0.3, prob.cens = 35%, $V \sim Unif(0, \sqrt{12})$, size = 1000 137

C.12.Boxplot for τ with beta.true = -0.2, tau.true = -0.3, prob.cens = 35%, $V \sim Unif(0, \sqrt{12})$, size = 1000 138

C.13.Boxplot for β_V with beta.true = 0.4, tau.true = 0.5, prob.cens = 0%, $V \sim N(0, 1)$, size = 100 140

C.14.Boxplot for τ with beta.true = 0.4, tau.true = 0.5 prob.cens = 0%, $V \sim N(0, 1)$, size = 100 141

C.15.Boxplot for β_V with beta.true = 0.4, tau.true = 0.5, prob.cens = 0%, $V \sim N(0, 1)$, size = 500 143

C.16.Boxplot for τ with beta.true = 0.4, tau.true = 0.5, prob.cens = 0%, $V \sim N(0, 1)$, size = 500 144

C.17.Boxplot for β_V with beta.true = 0.4, tau.true = 0.5, prob.cens = 0%, $V \sim N(0, 1)$, size = 1000 146

C.18.Boxplot for τ with beta.true = 0.4, tau.true = 0.5, prob.cens = 0%, $V \sim N(0, 1)$, size = 1000 147

C.19.Boxplot for β_V with beta.true = 0.4, tau.true = 0.5, prob.cens = 0%, $V \sim Unif(0, \sqrt{12})$, size = 100 149

C.20.Boxplot for τ with beta.true = 0.4, tau.true = 0.5, prob.cens = 0%, $V \sim Unif(0, \sqrt{12})$, size = 100 150

C.21.Boxplot for β_V with beta.true = 0.4, tau.true = 0.5, prob.cens = 0%, $V \sim Unif(0, \sqrt{12})$, size = 500 152

C.22.Boxplot for τ with beta.true = 0.4, tau.true = 0.5, prob.cens = 0%, $V \sim Unif(0, \sqrt{12})$, size = 500 153

C.23.Boxplot for β_V with beta.true = 0.4, tau.true = 0.5, prob.cens = 0%, $V \sim Unif(0, \sqrt{12})$, size = 1000 155

C.24.Boxplot for τ with beta.true = 0.4, tau.true = 0.5, prob.cens = 0%, $V \sim Unif(0, \sqrt{12})$, size = 1000 156

C.25.Boxplot for β_V with beta.V.true = 0.6, beta.F.true = -0.1, tau.true = -0.5, prob.cens = 0%, $V \sim N(0, 1)$, size = 100 158

C.26.Boxplot for β_F with beta.V.true = 0.6, beta.F.true = -0.1, tau.true = -0.5, prob.cens = 0%, $V \sim N(0, 1)$, size = 100 159

C.27. Boxplot for τ with beta.V.true $= 0.6$, beta.F.true $= -0.1$, tau.true
$= -0.5$, prob.cens $= 0\%$, $V \sim N(0,1)$, size $= 100$ 160

C.28. Boxplot for β_V with beta.V.true $= 0.6$, beta.F.true $= -0.1$, tau.true
$= -0.5$, prob.cens $= 0\%$, $V \sim N(0,1)$, size $= 500$ 163

C.29. Boxplot for β_F with beta.V.true $= 0.6$, beta.F.true $= -0.1$, tau.true
$= -0.5$, prob.cens $= 0\%$, $V \sim N(0,1)$, size $= 500$ 164

C.30. Boxplot for τ with beta.V.true $= 0.6$, beta.F.true $= -0.1$, tau.true
$= -0.5$, prob.cens $= 0\%$, $V \sim N(0,1)$, size $= 500$ 165

C.31. Boxplot for β_V with beta.V.true $= 0.6$, beta.F.true $= -0.1$, tau.true
$= -0.5$, prob.cens $= 0\%$, $V \sim N(0,1)$, size $= 1000$ 168

C.32. Boxplot for β_F with beta.V.true $= 0.6$, beta.F.true $= -0.1$, tau.true
$= -0.5$, prob.cens $= 0\%$, $V \sim N(0,1)$, size $= 1000$ 169

C.33. Boxplot for τ with beta.V.true $= 0.6$, beta.F.true $= -0.1$, tau.true
$= -0.5$, prob.cens $= 0\%$, $V \sim N(0,1)$, size $= 1000$ 170

C.34. Boxplot for β_V with beta.V.true $= 0.6$, beta.F.true $= -0.1$, tau.true
$= -0.5$, prob.cens $= 0\%$, $V \sim Unif(0, \sqrt{12})$, size $= 100$ 173

C.35. Boxplot for β_F with beta.V.true $= 0.6$, beta.F.true $= -0.1$, tau.true
$= -0.5$, prob.cens $= 0\%$, $V \sim Unif(0, \sqrt{12})$, size $= 100$ 174

C.36. Boxplot for τ with beta.V.true $= 0.6$, beta.F.true $= -0.1$, tau.true
$= -0.5$, prob.cens $= 0\%$, $V \sim Unif(0, \sqrt{12})$, size $= 100$ 175

C.37. Boxplot for β_V with beta.V.true $= 0.6$, beta.F.true $= -0.1$, tau.true
$= -0.5$, prob.cens $= 0\%$, $V \sim Unif(0, \sqrt{12})$, size $= 500$ 178

C.38. Boxplot for β_F with beta.V.true $= 0.6$, beta.F.true $= -0.1$, tau.true
$= -0.5$, prob.cens $= 0\%$, $V \sim Unif(0, \sqrt{12})$, size $= 500$ 179

C.39. Boxplot for τ with beta.V.true $= 0.6$, beta.F.true $= -0.1$, tau.true
$= -0.5$, prob.cens $= 0\%$, $V \sim Unif(0, \sqrt{12})$, size $= 500$ 180

C.40. Boxplot for β_V with beta.V.true $= 0.6$, beta.F.true $= -0.1$, tau.true
$= -0.5$, prob.cens $= 0\%$, $V \sim Unif(0, \sqrt{12})$, size $= 1000$ 183

C.41. Boxplot for β_F with beta.V.true $= 0.6$, beta.F.true $= -0.1$, tau.true
$= -0.5$, prob.cens $= 0\%$, $V \sim Unif(0, \sqrt{12})$, size $= 1000$ 184

C.42. Boxplot for τ with beta.V.true $= 0.6$, beta.F.true $= -0.1$, tau.true
$= -0.5$, prob.cens $= 0\%$, $V \sim Unif(0, \sqrt{12})$, size $= 1000$ 185

C.43. Boxplot for β_1 with beta.1.true $= 0.6$, beta.2.true $= -0.2$, tau.1.true
$= 0.5$, tau.2.true $= -0.4$, prob.cens $= 35\%$, $V \sim N(0,1)$, size $= 100$. 189

C.44. Boxplot for τ_1 with beta.1.true $= 0.6$, beta.2.true $= -0.2$, tau.1.true
$= 0.5$, tau.2.true $= -0.4$, prob.cens $= 35\%$, $V \sim N(0,1)$, size $= 100$. 190

C.45.Boxplot for β_2 with beta.1.true $= 0.6$, beta.2.true $= -0.2$, tau.1.true
$= 0.5$, tau.2.true $= -0.4$, prob.cens $= 35\%$, $V \sim N(0,1)$, size $= 100$. 191

C.46.Boxplot for τ_2 with beta.1.true $= 0.6$, beta.2.true $= -0.2$, tau.1.true
$= 0.5$, tau.2.true $= -0.4$, prob.cens $= 35\%$, $V \sim N(0,1)$, size $= 100$. 192

C.47.Boxplot for β_1 with beta.1.true $= 0.6$, beta.2.true $= -0.2$, tau.1.true
$= 0.5$, tau.2.true $= -0.4$, prob.cens $= 35\%$, $V \sim N(0,1)$, size $= 500$. 196

C.48.Boxplot for τ_1 with beta.1.true $= 0.6$, beta.2.true $= -0.2$, tau.1.true
$= 0.5$, tau.2.true $= -0.4$, prob.cens $= 35\%$, $V \sim N(0,1)$, size $= 500$. 197

C.49.Boxplot for β_2 with beta.1.true $= 0.6$, beta.2.true $= -0.2$, tau.1.true
$= 0.5$, tau.2.true $= -0.4$, prob.cens $= 35\%$, $V \sim N(0,1)$, size $= 500$. 198

C.50.Boxplot for τ_2 with beta.1.true $= 0.6$, beta.2.true $= -0.2$, tau.1.true
$= 0.5$, tau.2.true $= -0.4$, prob.cens $= 35\%$, $V \sim N(0,1)$, size $= 500$. 199

C.51.Boxplot for β_1 with beta.1.true $= 0.6$, beta.2.true $= -0.2$, tau.1.true
$= 0.5$, tau.2.true $= -0.4$, prob.cens $= 35\%$, $V \sim N(0,1)$, size $= 1000$ 203

C.52.Boxplot for τ_1 with beta.1.true $= 0.6$, beta.2.true $= -0.2$, tau.1.true
$= 0.5$, tau.2.true $= -0.4$, prob.cens $= 35\%$, $V \sim N(0,1)$, size $= 1000$ 204

C.53.Boxplot for β_2 with beta.1.true $= 0.6$, beta.2.true $= -0.2$, tau.1.true
$= 0.5$, tau.2.true $= -0.4$, prob.cens $= 35\%$, $V \sim N(0,1)$, size $= 1000$ 205

C.54.Boxplot for τ_2 with beta.1.true $= 0.6$, beta.2.true $= -0.2$, tau.1.true
$= 0.5$, tau.2.true $= -0.4$, prob.cens $= 35\%$, $V \sim N(0,1)$, size $= 1000$ 206

C.55.Boxplot for beta.1.true $= 0.6$, beta.2.true $= -0.2$, tau.1.true $= 0.5$,
tau.2.true $= -0.4$, prob.cens $= 0\%$ and $V \sim N(0,1)$, size $= 100$, sd.U
$= 0$ and sd.U $= 0.1$ 225

C.56.Boxplot for beta.1.true $= 0.6$, beta.2.true $= -0.2$, tau.1.true $= 0.5$,
tau.2.true $= -0.4$, prob.cens $= 0\%$ and $V \sim N(0,1)$, size $= 100$, sd.U
$= 0.4$ and sd.U $= 0.8$ 226

C.57.Boxplot for beta.1.true $= 0.6$, beta.2.true $= -0.2$, tau.1.true $= 0.5$,
tau.2.true $= -0.4$, prob.cens $= 0\%$ and $V \sim N(0,1)$, size $= 500$, sd.U
$= 0$ and sd.U $= 0.1$ 227

C.58.Boxplot for beta.1.true $= 0.6$, beta.2.true $= -0.2$, tau.1.true $= 0.5$,
tau.2.true $= -0.4$, prob.cens $= 0\%$ and $V \sim N(0,1)$, size $= 500$, sd.U
$= 0.4$ and sd.U $= 0.8$ 228

C.59.Boxplot for beta.1.true $= 0.6$, beta.2.true $= -0.2$, tau.1.true $= 0.5$,
tau.2.true $= -0.4$, prob.cens $= 0\%$ and $V \sim N(0,1)$, size $= 1000$,
sd.U $= 0$ and sd.U $= 0.1$ 229

C.60. Boxplot for `beta.1.true` = 0.6, `beta.2.true` = -0.2 , `tau.1.true` = 0.5, `tau.2.true` = -0.4, `prob.cens` = 0% and $V \sim N(0,1)$, `size` = 1000, `sd.U` = 0.4 and `sd.U` = 0.8 230

List of Tables

4.1. Simulation grid for *Check the fit Function* with $\tilde{Y} \sim W$ and `monte.carlo` $= 1000$ 59

4.2. Simulation grid for *Check the fit Function* with $\tilde{Y} \sim W + F$ and `monte.carlo` $= 1000$ 67

4.3. Simulation grid for *Structural Changes* with $\tilde{Y} \sim W \mid Z_1$ and `monte.carlo` $= 500$ 75

4.4. Simulation grid for *Structural Changes* with $\tilde{Y} \sim W \mid Z_1 + Z_2$ and `monte.carlo` $= 500$ 83

C.1. Results for β_V and τ with `beta.true` $= -0.2$, `tau.true` $= -0.3$, `prob.cens` $= 35\%$, $V \sim N(0,1)$ and `size` $= 100$ 124

C.2. Results for β_V and τ with `beta.true` $= -0.2$, `tau.true` $= -0.3$, `prob.cens` $= 35\%$, $V \sim N(0,1)$ and `size` $= 500$ 127

C.3. Results for β_V and τ with `beta.true` $= -0.2$, `tau.true` $= -0.3$, `prob.cens` $= 35\%$, $V \sim N(0,1)$ and `size` $= 1000$ 130

C.4. Results for β_V and τ with `beta.true` $= -0.2$, `tau.true` $= -0.3$, `prob.cens` $= 35\%$, $V \sim Unif(0, \sqrt{12})$ and `size` $= 100$ 133

C.5. Results for β_V and τ with `beta.true` $= -0.2$, `tau.true` $= -0.3$, `prob.cens` $= 35\%$, $V \sim Unif(0, \sqrt{12})$ and `size` $= 500$ 136

C.6. Results for β_V and τ with `beta.true` $= -0.2$, `tau.true` $= -0.3$, `prob.cens` $= 35\%$, $V \sim Unif(0, \sqrt{12})$ and `size` $= 1000$ 139

C.7. Results for β_V and τ with `beta.true` $= 0.4$, `tau.true` $= 0.5$, `prob.cens` $= 0\%$, $V \sim N(0,1)$ and `size` $= 100$ 142

C.8. Results for β_V and τ with `beta.true` $= 0.4$, `tau.true` $= 0.5$, `prob.cens` $= 0\%$, $V \sim N(0,1)$ and `size` $= 500$ 145

C.9. Results for β_V and τ with `beta.true` $= 0.4$, `tau.true` $= 0.5$, `prob.cens` $= 0\%$, $V \sim N(0,1)$ and `size` $= 1000$ 148

C.10.Results for β_V and τ with `beta.true` $= 0.4$, `tau.true` $= 0.5$, `prob.cens` $= 0\%$, $V \sim Unif(0, \sqrt{12})$ and `size` $= 100$ 151

C.11.Results for β_V and τ with beta.true = 0.4, tau.true = 0.5, prob.cens = 0%, $V \sim Unif(0, \sqrt{12})$ and size = 500 154

C.12.Results for β_V and τ with beta.true = 0.4, tau.true = 0.5, prob.cens = 0%, $V \sim Unif(0, \sqrt{12})$ and size = 1000 157

C.13.Results for β_V and β_F with beta.V.true = 0.6, beta.F.true = -0.1, tau.true = -0.5, prob.cens = 0%, $V \sim N(0, 1)$ and size = 100 161

C.14.Results for τ with beta.V.true = 0.6, beta.F.true = -0.1, tau.true = -0.5, prob.cens = 0%, $V \sim N(0, 1)$ and size = 100 162

C.15.Results for β_V and β_F with beta.V.true = 0.6, beta.F.true = -0.1, tau.true = -0.5, prob.cens = 0%, $V \sim N(0, 1)$ and size = 500 166

C.16.Results for τ with beta.V.true = 0.6, beta.F.true = -0.1, tau.true = -0.5, prob.cens = 0%, $V \sim N(0, 1)$ and size = 500 167

C.17.Results for β_V and β_F with beta.V.true = 0.6, beta.F.true = -0.1, tau.true = -0.5, prob.cens = 0%, $V \sim N(0, 1)$ and size = 1000 171

C.18.Results for τ with beta.V.true = 0.6, beta.F.true = -0.1, tau.true = -0.5, prob.cens = 0%, $V \sim N(0, 1)$ and size = 1000 172

C.19.Results for β_V and β_F with beta.V.true = 0.6, beta.F.true = -0.1, tau.true = -0.5, prob.cens = 0%, $V \sim Unif(0, \sqrt{12})$ and size = 100 . 176

C.20.Results for τ with beta.V.true = 0.6, beta.F.true = -0.1, tau.true = -0.5, prob.cens = 0%, $V \sim Unif(0, \sqrt{12})$ and size = 100 177

C.21.Results for β_V and β_F with beta.V.true = 0.6, beta.F.true = -0.1, tau.true = -0.5, prob.cens = 0%, $V \sim Unif(0, \sqrt{12})$ and size = 500 . 181

C.22.Results for τ with beta.V.true = 0.6, beta.F.true = -0.1, tau.true = -0.5, prob.cens = 0%, $V \sim Unif(0, \sqrt{12})$ and size = 500 182

C.23.Results for β_V and β_F with beta.V.true = 0.6, beta.F.true = -0.1, tau.true = -0.5, prob.cens = 0%, $V \sim Unif(0, \sqrt{12})$ and size = 1000 186

C.24.Results for τ with beta.V.true = 0.6, beta.F.true = -0.1, tau.true = -0.5, prob.cens = 0%, $V \sim Unif(0, \sqrt{12})$ and size = 1000 187

C.25.Detection of the true structural change with beta.1.true = 0.6, beta.2.true = -0.2 , tau.1.true = 0.5, tau.2.true = -0.4, prob.cens = 35%, $V \sim N(0, 1)$ and size = 100 188

C.26.Results for node 2 with beta.1.true = 0.6, beta.2.true = -0.2 , tau.1.true = 0.5, tau.2.true = -0.4, prob.cens = 35%, $V \sim N(0, 1)$ and size = 100 193

C.27.Results for node 3 with `beta.1.true` = 0.6, `beta.2.true` = -0.2 , `tau.1.true` = 0.5, `tau.2.true` = -0.4, `prob.cens` = 35%, $V \sim N(0,1)$ and `size` = 100 194

C.28.Detection of the true structural change with `beta.1.true` = 0.6, `beta.2.true` = -0.2 , `tau.1.true` = 0.5, `tau.2.true` = -0.4, `prob.cens` = 35%, $V \sim N(0,1)$ and `size` = 500 195

C.29.Results for node 2 with `beta.1.true` = 0.6, `beta.2.true` = -0.2 , `tau.1.true` = 0.5, `tau.2.true` = -0.4, `prob.cens` = 35%, $V \sim N(0,1)$ and `size` = 500 200

C.30.Results for node 3 with `beta.1.true` = 0.6, `beta.2.true` = -0.2 , `tau.1.true` = 0.5, `tau.2.true` = -0.4, `prob.cens` = 35%, $V \sim N(0,1)$ and `size` = 500 201

C.31.Detection of the true structural change with `beta.1.true` = 0.6, `beta.2.true` = -0.2 , `tau.1.true` = 0.5, `tau.2.true` = -0.4, `prob.cens` = 35%, $V \sim N(0,1)$ and `size` = 1000 202

C.32.Results for node 2 with `beta.1.true` = 0.6, `beta.2.true` = -0.2 , `tau.1.true` = 0.5, `tau.2.true` = -0.4, `prob.cens` = 35%, $V \sim N(0,1)$ and `size` = 1000 207

C.33.Results for node 3 with `beta.1.true` = 0.6, `beta.2.true` = -0.2 , `tau.1.true` = 0.5, `tau.2.true` = -0.4, `prob.cens` = 35%, $V \sim N(0,1)$ and `size` = 1000 208

C.34.Detection of the true structural changes with `beta.1.true` = -0.9, `beta.2.true` = 0.2 , `beta.3.true` = 1.1, `tau.1.true` = 0.5, `tau.2.true` = 0.5, `tau.3.true` = 0.5, `prob.cens` = 0%, $V \sim N(0,1)$ and `size` = 100, 500, 1000 209

C.35.Detection of the true structural changes with `beta.1.true` = -0.9, `beta.2.true` = 0.2 , `beta.3.true` = 1.1, `tau.1.true` = 0.5, `tau.2.true` = 0.5, `tau.3.true` = 0.5, `prob.cens` = 35%, $V \sim N(0,1)$ and `size` = 100, 500, 1000 210

C.36.Detection of the true structural changes with `beta.1.true` = -0.9, `beta.2.true` = 0.2 , `beta.3.true` = 1.1, `tau.1.true` = 0.5, `tau.2.true` = 0.5, `tau.3.true` = 0.5, `prob.cens` = 65%, $V \sim N(0,1)$ and `size` = 100, 500, 1000 211

C.37.Detection of the true structural changes with `beta.1.true` = 0.4, `beta.2.true` = 0.4, `beta.3.true` = 0.4, `tau.1.true` = -1, `tau.2.true` = 0.1, `tau.3.true` = 0.9, `prob.cens` = 0%, $V \sim N(0,1)$ and `size` = 100, 500, 1000 212

C.38. Detection of the true structural changes with beta.1.true = 0.4, beta.2.true
= 0.4 , beta.3.true = 0.4, tau.1.true = -1, tau.2.true = 0.1, tau.3.true
= 0.9, prob.cens = 35%, $V \sim N(0,1)$ and size = 100, 500, 1000 213

C.39. Detection of the true structural changes with beta.1.true = 0.4, beta.2.true
= 0.4 , beta.3.true = 0.4, tau.1.true = -1, tau.2.true = 0.1, tau.3.true
= 0.9, prob.cens = 65%, $V \sim N(0,1)$ and size = 100, 500, 1000 214

C.40. Detection of the true structural changes with beta.1.true = -0.9, beta.2.true
= 0.2 , beta.3.true = 1.1, tau.1.true = -1, tau.2.true = 0.1, tau.3.true
= 0.9, prob.cens = 0%, $V \sim N(0,1)$ and size = 100, 500, 1000 215

C.41. Detection of the true structural changes with beta.1.true = -0.9, beta.2.true
= 0.2 , beta.3.true = 1.1, tau.1.true = -1, tau.2.true = 0.1, tau.3.true
= 0.9, prob.cens = 35%, $V \sim N(0,1)$ and size = 100, 500, 1000 216

C.42. Detection of the true structural changes with beta.1.true = -0.9, beta.2.true
= 0.2 , beta.3.true = 1.1, tau.1.true = -1, tau.2.true = 0.1, tau.3.true
= 0.9, prob.cens = 65%, $V \sim N(0,1)$ and size = 100, 500, 1000 217

C.43. Prediction error with 95% confidence interval with beta.1.true = 0.6,
beta.2.true = -0.2 , tau.1.true = 0.5, tau.2.true = -0.4, prob.cens
= 0%, $V \sim N(0,1)$ and size = 100 231

C.44. Prediction error with 95% confidence interval with beta.1.true = 0.6,
beta.2.true = -0.2 , tau.1.true = 0.5, tau.2.true = -0.4, prob.cens
= 0%, $V \sim N(0,1)$ and size = 500 232

C.45. Prediction error with 95% confidence interval with beta.1.true = 0.6,
beta.2.true = -0.2 , tau.1.true = 0.5, tau.2.true = -0.4, prob.cens
= 0%, $V \sim N(0,1)$ and size = 1000 233

1. Introduction

The model-based recursive partitioning (MOB), which was developed by Zeileis et al. (2008), to analyse the influence of independent covariables on an outcome variable provides an alternative to standard multiple regression models. The algorithmic method is a combination of non-parametric classification trees and parametric models and is therefore a semi-parametric approach. Here, the Cox's proportional hazards model (Cox, 1972) (in the following only referred to as Cox model), which has been established as the most popular regression model for analysing time-to-event data, is considered. The analysis of time-to-event data is employed in different areas of application, such as in medical sciences, sociology, psychology, econometrics and political sciences. The focus of the thesis is on medical sciences. Particularly, in biometric studies covariables of interest can often not be recorded exactly, therefore surrogates have to be used instead. The resulting naive estimation, ignoring the measurement error, leads to biased estimators. For statistical models including covariates which are subject to measurement errors, also termed as error-in-variables models, several methods exit to adjust for the measurement error. The methods can be divided into structural and functional approaches. For example, a simple approach is the regression calibration, which is easy to implement. Here, a functional approach is considered, based on the methodology of the corrected score function. Motivated by the suggested approach of Nakamura (1992) under the assumption of an additive measurement error model, Augustin (2004) suggested a corrected score function for the Cox model, which integrates an adjustment for measurement error in the so-called Breslow likelihood (Breslow, 1972, 1974). In addition, the corrected score function is extended for more than one error-prone covariable and for error-free covariables. The suggested concept can also be applied to a form of regression models, where the hazard rate is parameterised, here the Weibull model is considered.

In this thesis an adjustment for measurement error in the Cox and Weibull model is incorporated theoretically in the framework of the model-based recursive partitioning, which was to the author's knowledge not examined so far. Therefore, the corrected score functions are integrated into the algorithm of the model-based recursive partitioning that relies on score functions.

In the R package party (Hothorn et al., 2010) a function mob() (Zeileis et al., 2008) is available to conduct model-based recursive partitioning. A model-based parameter estimation is already integrated for the Weibull model. The main challenge is to extend the implemented estimation for the Weibull model with measurement error correction. This means that here the focus is set to the Weibull model. For the implementation of the underlying problem, R version 2.11.1 (R Development Core Team, 2010) is used.

The remainder of the thesis is organized as follows: In Chapter 2, first the theoretical background of the Cox and Weibull model is described. The concept of the corrected score function to adjust for measurement error is integrated in the framework of the Cox and Weibull model under the assumption of an additive measurement error model. A short introduction to classification trees and regression trees is given to motivate the concept of model-based recursive partitioning. Furthermore, the algorithm of the model-based recursive partitioning is described. By the integration of the corrected parameter estimation in the Cox and Weibull model the two topics are brought together. In Chapter 3, the implementation of the corrected MOB algorithm, which integrates the corrected score functions of the Weibull model, is presented. In Chapter 4, the implementation is validated on the basis of a simulation study by comparing the performance of the new implemented corrected parameter estimation to a benchmark estimation, a naive estimation and a corrected parameter estimation obtained by the regression calibration.

2. Theoretical Background

2.1. Cox Model and Measurement Error

In biometric studies the Cox's *proportional hazards model* (Cox, 1972) has been established as the most popular regression model for analysing survival data. This kind of data is characterized by two parts. On the one hand by *failure*, which describes the occurrence of an event such as death or a specific disease, and on the other hand by *failure time*, which is the time period until the event occurs. A special property of survival data is the presence of *censoring*. A subject is called as censored, when it drops out early without having an event or is event free by the end of the study. This type of censorship is also called *right censoring*. Here, only this type of censorship is considered. For a detailed overview of the different censoring mechanisms see e. g. Kalbfleisch and Prentice (2002).

More formally the survival data for a subject i, $i = 1, \ldots, n$, is defined as follows: T_i denotes the failure time and δ_i is an indicator function, which is 1 if the subject has an event and 0 if the subject is censored. The pair (Y_i, δ_i) characterizes the survival data, where $Y_i = min(T_i, C_i)$ and C_i is the censoring time. The censoring process is assumed to be stochastically independent of T_i given the covariates V_i. The Cox model is used to explore the effect of the covariables on the censored failure times. For example, a question of interest could be how smoking affects the appearance of lung cancer. Before the definition of the Cox model is specified, a few fundamental definitions have to be outlined. A central concept to interpret the Cox model is the *hazard rate* $h(t)$, which is based on the conditional probability that an event occurs in the interval $[t, t + \Delta t)$, given the subject has reached the interval. It is defined by

$$h(t) = \lim_{\Delta t \to 0} \frac{P(t \leq T < t + \Delta t | T \geq t)}{\Delta t} = \frac{f(t)}{S(t)}, \tag{2.1}$$

where t is an arbitrary point in time and T the failure time. The hazard rate can also be described by the ratio of the density function $f(t)$ and the survival function $S(t) = P(T \geq t)$ of T. The density function $f(t)$ is equal to the derivative of the distribution function $F(t) = P(T < t)$. $F(t)$ denotes the probability for the occurrence of an event (before t). The *survival function* is the inverse of $F(t)$, thus $S(t)$ is also given by $S(t) = 1 - F(t)$ and describes the probability that no event has occurred before t or in other words the probability to survive the time point t. From the hazard rate the *cumulative hazard rate* is derived:

$$H(t) = \int_0^t h(u)du = \int_0^t \frac{f(u)}{S(u)}du = -ln(S(t)), \tag{2.2}$$

which is the cumulative risk for an event over the time. Therefore, the survival function is also characterized via the cumulative hazard rate, $S(t) = exp(-H(t))$. In the Cox model the hazard rate is considered as a function of the covariates. The model is given for subject i, $i = 1, \dots, n$, with a vector of covariates V_i by

$$h(t, V_i) = h_0(t) \cdot exp(V_i' \beta), \tag{2.3}$$

where β is the unknown coefficient vector for V_i. $h_0(t)$ denotes the *baseline hazard* and specifies the risk for an event in t given all covariates are set to zero. The baseline hazard can be left unspecified. Thus, the model is a semi-parametric approach, i. e. no assumption about the distribution of the hazard rate is made, and therefore quite flexible in practice. The Cox model underlies the so-called *proportional hazard assumption*. The ratio of the hazard function of subject i with a set of covariates V_i and a subject j with a set of covariates V_j is equal to

$$\frac{h(t, V_i)}{h(t, V_j)} = \frac{h_0(t) \cdot exp(V_i' \beta)}{h_0(t) \cdot exp(V_j' \beta)} = exp([V_i - V_j]\beta) = const. \tag{2.4}$$

The ratio does not depend on t, i. e. the effect of the covariates on the hazard rate is proportional over the time. The ratio is also called *hazard ratio*.

Given that $h_0(t)$ is not specified, it is not possible to conduct a usual likelihood estimation for β. A so-called *partial likelihood* is employed, where $h_0(t)$ is considered as a nuisance parameter. The root of the derivative of the partial log-likelihood

$$\sum_{j=1}^k \left(V_j - \frac{\sum_{i \in R(\pi_j)} V_i \cdot exp(\beta' V_i)}{\sum_{i \in R(\pi_j)} exp(\beta' V_i)} \right) = 0, \tag{2.5}$$

provides the parameter estimation $\hat{\beta}$ (more details in Section 2.1.3).

Often in medical surveys covariates of interest cannot be recorded exactly. Surrogates have to be used instead. For example, the true blood pressure is difficult to investigate, usually an average over frequent measurements is taken. By using the surrogates W_i instead of V_i the naive estimator $\hat{\beta}_{naive}$ of β is obtained by maximizing the likelihood function. Substituting V_i by W_i in the score function of the Cox model result in

$$\sum_{j=1}^{k} \left(W_j - \frac{\sum_{i \in R(\pi_j)} W_i \cdot exp(\beta' W_i)}{\sum_{i \in R(\pi_j)} exp(\beta' W_i)} \right) = 0. \tag{2.6}$$

The root of this so-called *naive score function* is the naive parameter estimator $\hat{\beta}_{naive}$. Ignoring the measurement error, $\hat{\beta}_{naive}$ is biased and does not converge to the true parameter, as has been illustrated by Prentice (1982). Statistical models, including covariates which are subject to measurement errors, also termed as *error-in-variables models*. For this model class several methods exit to adjust for error in variables (see Section 2.1.2). A detailed description is given in Carroll et al. (2006).

2.1.1. Measurement Error Model

The adjustment for measurement errors is only possible due to the knowledge of the relationship between the true variables V_i and the surrogates W_i. An *additive measurement error model* (Carroll et al., 2006, Chapter 1) is assumed:

$$W_i = V_i + U_i, \tag{2.7}$$

with $\mathbb{E}(U_i) = 0$, $i = 1, \ldots, n$, and U_i is independent of V_i, T_i, δ_i, and of U_l ($l \neq i$), i. e. the errors U_i are taken to be independent among each other. Furthermore, the distribution of the measurement error U_i has to be known. An identically distribution is not necessary, so that heteroscedastic or homoscedastic errors can be considered. The *moment generating function* of the specified distribution has to exist for all a and is defined by

$$M_{U_i}(a) = \mathbb{E}(exp(a' U_i)), \tag{2.8}$$

which is twice differentiable with respect to a. $M_{U_i}(\cdot)$ is required for the correction of the likelihood and accordingly of the score function (see Section 2.1.3). The outcome variable T_i and δ_i are assumed to be error free. The covariates are independent of time and the variables measured with error are taken to be continuous.

2.1.2. Adjustment for Measurement Error in Cox Model

Several authors have dealt with the question how to adjust for measurement error in the Cox model (e. g. Prentice, 1982; Wang et al., 1997; Buzas, 1998; Hu et al., 1998; Kong et al., 1998; Nakamura, 1992; Augustin, 2004), an overview is given in Augustin and Schwarz (2002). Moreover, Huang and Wang (2000); Hu and Lin (2002); Gorfine et al. (2004); Liu et al. (2004); Li and Ryan (2006); Yi and Lawless (2007); Zucker and Spiegelman (2008) and Wen (2009) have concentrated on this subject.

For the inference on the regression coefficients β, there are two kinds of measurement error models, the *functional* and the *structural approach* (Carroll et al., 2006, Chapter 2). The main difference between these two approaches is the assumption about the distribution of true variables V_i. In the structural method the distribution of V_i is taken to follow a known class of distributions. The functional approach gets along without any parametric assumption on the distribution of V_i.

Structural Approach

The two basic approaches are *regression calibration* and *integrating the likelihood*, where the measurement error is assumed to be homoscedastic. In the following only the regression calibration is outlined, which is used as a comparison to the new implemented approach in the simulation study (see Chapter 4). The basis of the regression calibration is to replace the true but unobservable variables V_i by the regression of V_i on W_i. For inference on β via the likelihood the conditional expectation $\mathbb{E}(V_i|W_i)$ is used instead of V_i. Assuming that V_i is i.i.d. normally distributed with unknown mean μ_V and non-singular covariance matrix Σ_V. Then $W_i \sim N(\mu_V; \Sigma_V + \Sigma_U)$ and $V_i|W_i \sim N(\bar{\mu}_i, \bar{\Sigma})$. Σ_U is an estimator of the measurement error covariance matrix, usually derived from validation data or repeated measurements. In addition, a low failure rate is assumed, also named as *rare disease assumption*. The conditional expectation $\mathbb{E}(V_i|W_i)$ is given by

$$\bar{\mu}_i = \mu_V + \Sigma_V \cdot (\Sigma_V + \Sigma_U)^{-1} \cdot (W_i - \mu_V) \tag{2.9}$$

and $\bar{\Sigma} = \Sigma_V - \Sigma_V \cdot (\Sigma_V + \Sigma_U)^{-1}$ (Augustin and Schwarz, 2002). The estimated conditional expectation is computed as follows

$$\hat{\bar{\mu}}_i = \hat{\mu}_W + (\hat{\Sigma}_W - \hat{\Sigma}_U) \cdot (\hat{\Sigma}_W)^{-1} \cdot (W_i - \hat{\mu}_W), \qquad (2.10)$$

given that under the additive measurement error model $\mu_W = \mu_V + \mu_U$ and $\mu_U = 0$ as well as $\Sigma_W = \Sigma_V + \Sigma_U \Leftrightarrow \Sigma_V = \Sigma_W - \Sigma_U$.

Replacing V_i by the conditional expectation $\bar{\mu}_i$ in Equation (2.5) leads to

$$\sum_{j=1}^{k} \left(\bar{\mu}_i - \frac{\sum_{i \in R(\pi_j)} \bar{\mu}_i \cdot exp(\beta' \bar{\mu}_i)}{\sum_{i \in R(\pi_j)} exp(\beta' \bar{\mu}_i)} \right) = 0. \qquad (2.11)$$

It can be shown that the corrected parameter estimation $\hat{\beta}_{corr}$ is equal to $\Sigma_V^{-1} \cdot (\Sigma_V + \Sigma_U) \cdot \hat{\beta}_{naive}$. This estimator corresponds to the method in the linear model by multiplying $\hat{\beta}$ with the inverse reliability ratio (see Carroll et al., 2006, Chapter 3). The adjusted estimates are not necessarily consistent, but the bias reduction is substantial (Augustin and Schwarz, 2002). In addition, the approach is easy to implement. Wang et al. (1997) derive this approach for the Cox model in a functional way, where the estimation of the distribution of $V_i|W_i$ is carried out via validation data.

Functional Approach

An established procedure is suggested by Nakamura (1992), which is based on the methodology of the *corrected score function* (see Nakamura, 1990; Carroll et al., 2006, Chapter 7). A corrected score function is proposed, which leads to approximately unbiased estimates. For the correction no distribution assumptions have to be made about the covariates V_i.

In general, a corrected score function to estimate the parameter vector ϑ is one whose conditional expectation with respect to the measurement error distribution coincides with the usual score function based on the unknown true variables V_i (Nakamura, 1990)(see Equation (2.12) below). Given is the sample $\tilde{Y} = (\tilde{Y}_1, \ldots, \tilde{Y}_n)$ with covariates $V = (V_1, \ldots, V_n)$ and surrogates $W = (W_1, \ldots, W_n)$. $s^V(\tilde{Y}, V, \vartheta)$ denotes the *ideal score function*, since V is unobservable. Replacing V by W yields to the *naive score function* $s^V(\tilde{Y}, W, \vartheta)$. In general, $\mathbb{E}_{\vartheta_0}(s^V(\tilde{Y}, W, \vartheta_0))$, where ϑ_0 is the true parameter value of ϑ, is not equal to zero and therefore the naive score function leads to a biased estimator of ϑ. The main idea is to find a corrected score function $s^W(\tilde{Y}, W, \vartheta)$ and the corrected log-likelihood $l^W(\tilde{Y}, W, \vartheta)$, respectively, such that

$$\mathbb{E}_\vartheta(s^W(\tilde{Y}, W, \vartheta|V, \tilde{Y})) = s^V(\tilde{Y}, V, \vartheta) \tag{2.12}$$

$$\mathbb{E}_\vartheta(l^W(\tilde{Y}, W, \vartheta|V, \tilde{Y})) = l^V(\tilde{Y}, V, \vartheta) \tag{2.13}$$

$$\text{with } s^W(\tilde{Y}, W, \vartheta) := \frac{\partial}{\partial \vartheta} l^W(\tilde{Y}, W, \vartheta) \ \forall \vartheta. \tag{2.14}$$

In addition, $\mathbb{E}_{\vartheta_0}(s^V(\tilde{Y}, V, \vartheta_0)) = 0$ holds, thus by the law of iterated expectation

$$\mathbb{E}_{\vartheta_0}(s^W(\tilde{Y}, W, \vartheta_0)) = \mathbb{E}_{\vartheta_0}(\mathbb{E}_{\vartheta_0}(s^W(\tilde{Y}, W, \vartheta_0|V, \tilde{Y}))) = \mathbb{E}_{\vartheta_0}(s^V(\tilde{Y}, V, \vartheta_0)) = 0. \tag{2.15}$$

The estimator $\hat{\vartheta}$ obtained by solving $s^W(\tilde{Y}, W, \hat{\vartheta}) = 0$, such that $-\partial s^W(\tilde{Y}, W, \hat{\vartheta})/\partial \vartheta$ is positive definite, is called the corrected estimator for ϑ. Given ϑ is of finite dimension, under certain regularity conditions $\hat{\vartheta}$ is a consistent and asymptotically normal estimator of ϑ (Nakamura, 1990; Carroll et al., 2006, Appendix A.6). M-estimation techniques for the calculation of standard errors and for inference on $\hat{\vartheta}$ are used (Carroll et al., 2006, Chapter 7).

Stefanski (1989) shows that the concept of the corrected score function cannot be applied to the usual likelihood inference for the Cox model. The denominator of the partial estimation function in Equation (2.5) shows a (complex) singularity, thus an exact correction of the partial likelihood does not exist (Nakamura, 1992; Augustin and Schwarz, 2002). Therefore, Nakamura (1992) suggests an adjustment via a first and second order Taylor approximation under the assumption of homoscedastic normal measurement error. Kong and Gu (1999) show that the estimator suggested by Nakamura (1992) is consistent and has an asymptotic normal distribution. Kong et al. (1998) derive the corresponding corrected estimator of the cumulative baseline hazard rate. An extension to homoscedastic non-normal error is captured in Kong and Gu (1999).

Augustin (2004) shows that the concept of the first order estimator by Nakamura (1992) and the corrected baseline hazard rate estimator by Kong et al. (1998) can be applied to the *Breslow likelihood* (Breslow, 1972, 1974). An exact corrected likelihood approach is derived, which allows to estimate a corrected version of the regression coefficients β and the cumulative baseline hazard under heteroscedastic and non-normal measurement error. The suggested concept can also be applied to a form of regression models, where the hazard rate is parameterised, e. g. the Weibull model. The focus in the master's thesis is on the approach suggested by

Augustin (2004) and is described in the next section in detail. In addition, the corrected log-likelihood is extended for more than one error-prone covariate and for error-free covariables.

2.1.3. Corrected Log-Likelihood and Score Function in Cox and Weibull Model

Let $Y_i = min(T_i, C_i)$, $i = 1, \ldots, n$, be the censored failure times and δ_i be the indicator function for censoring. Let $\pi_1 < \pi_2 < \ldots < \pi_k$ be the different ordered failure times and be $d_j := |D_j(\pi_j)|$, $j = 1, \ldots, k$, the number of all subjects, which failed at π_j. If d_j is greater than 1, so-called *ties* exist in the data set. This means that more than one event occur at the same time. In such cases, the partial likelihood has to be corrected. Different methods exist to adjust for ties, here the correction by Peto (1972) and Breslow (1974) is considered, see Equation (2.18). $R(\pi_j)$ denotes the *risk set*, which includes all subjects, which are alive immediately before $\pi_j, j = 0, 1, \ldots, k, \pi_0 := 0$. A set of covariates is considered, which consists of covariates measured with and without error. Let $A_i = \begin{pmatrix} W_i \\ F_i \end{pmatrix}$ be the observed covariates vector, which consists of W_i subject to measurement error and underlie an additive error model from Equation (2.7) $W_i = V_i + U_i$ with $U_i \perp \{V_i, T_i, \delta_i\}$ and $U_i \perp U_l$ $(i \neq l)$, as well as F_i, which are free of measurement error. Let $X_i = \begin{pmatrix} V_i \\ F_i \end{pmatrix}$, which includes the true but unobservable covariables V_i. In matrix notation the design matrix is given by

$$
X = \underbrace{\begin{pmatrix} 1 & V_{11} & \cdots & V_{1p} & F_{1p+1} & \cdots & F_{1m} \\ \vdots & \vdots & & \vdots & \vdots & & \vdots \\ 1 & V_{i1} & \cdots & V_{ip} & F_{ip+1} & \cdots & F_{im} \\ \vdots & \vdots & & \vdots & \vdots & & \vdots \\ 1 & V_{n1} & \cdots & V_{np} & F_{np+1} & \cdots & F_{nm} \end{pmatrix}}_{(n \times m+1)} \text{ and } X_i = \underbrace{\begin{pmatrix} 1 \\ V_{i1} \\ \vdots \\ V_{ip} \\ F_{ip+1} \\ \vdots \\ F_{im} \end{pmatrix}}_{(m+1 \times 1)}, \quad (2.16)
$$

with m = number of covariates and n = number of observations.

The adjustment for measurement error via the moment generating function $M_{U_i}(\beta_X)$ is only required for the error-prone variables W_J, $J = 1, \ldots, p$. For the error-free variables F_J, $J = p+1, \ldots, m$, the moment generating function is set to 1. β_X is a $(m+1)$-dimensional vector defined as follows

$$\beta_X = (\beta_0, \beta_{V_1}, \cdots, \beta_{V_p}, \beta_{F_{p+1}}, \cdots, \beta_{F_m})'. \tag{2.17}$$

In the case of the Cox model, X is defined without the column with 1s, X_i without the row with 1 and β_X without the intercept β_0, because the Cox model includes the intercept via the baseline hazard rate.

Cox Model

In Cox (1972, 1975) an estimation of the parameter vector β by maximizing the partial likelihood is suggested and is given by

$$L^X(\pi, X, \beta_X) = \prod_{j=1}^{k} \left(\frac{exp(\beta_X' X_j)}{\left[\sum_{i \in R(\pi_j)} exp(\beta_X' X_i) \right]^{d_j}} \right)^{\delta_j}, \tag{2.18}$$

where $\pi = (\pi_1, \ldots, \pi_k)$ and a correction for ties by Peto (1972) and Breslow (1974) is included. From the log-likelihood

$$l^X(\pi, X, \beta_X) = \sum_{j=1}^{k} \left[\sum_{i \in D(\pi_j)} \beta_X' X_i - d_j \cdot ln \left[\sum_{i \in R(\pi_j)} exp(\beta_X' X_i) \right] \right] \tag{2.19}$$

the estimation equation is derived as

$$s^X(\pi, X, \beta_X) = \sum_{j=1}^{k} \left[\sum_{i \in D(\pi_j)} X_i - d_j \cdot \frac{\sum_{i \in R(\pi_j)} X_i \cdot exp(\beta_X' X_i)}{\sum_{i \in R(\pi_j)} exp(\beta_X' X_i)} \right] = 0, \tag{2.20}$$

which is equal to Equation (2.5), besides the correction for ties. For inference on the baseline hazard rate $h_0(t)$ the *Breslow estimator* (Breslow, 1972, 1974) of the cumulative baseline hazard

$$\hat{H}_0^{Br}(t) = \sum_{j:\pi_j \leq t} \frac{d_j}{\sum_{i \in R(\pi_j)} exp(\hat{\beta}_X' X_i)} \tag{2.21}$$

with $H_0(t) = \int_0^t h_0(u)du$ is considered.

As already mentioned, the concept of corrected score function cannot be applied to the score function derived by the partial log-likelihood in Equation (2.20). Thus

Augustin (2004) used the *Breslow likelihood* for derivation of a corrected parameter estimator for β instead. The *Breslow likelihood* was developed by Breslow (1972, 1974) to justify the partial likelihood (2.18) and to obtain the baseline hazard estimator from Equation (2.21).

Assuming piecewise constant hazard rate $h_0(t) \equiv h_j > 0, \pi_{j-1} < t < \pi_j, j = 1, \ldots, k$, the Breslow likelihood and log-likelihood is given, respectively, by

$$L_{Br}^X(\pi, X, \beta_X, h_j) = \prod_{i=1}^{n} \left[\left(h_0(t_i) exp(\beta_X' X_i) \right)^{\delta_i} exp \left(-exp(\beta_X' X_i) \cdot \int_0^{t_i} h_0(u) du \right) \right],$$

$$(2.22)$$

$$l_{Br}^X(\pi, X, \beta_X, h_j) = \sum_{j=1}^{k} \left[d_j ln(h_j) + \sum_{i \in D(\pi_j)} \beta_X' X_i - h_j(\pi_j - \pi_{j-1}) \sum_{i \in R(\pi_j)} exp(\beta_X' X_i) \right]$$

$$(2.23)$$

Corrected Log-Likelihood and Score Function of the Cox Model

Equation (2.23) does not possess any singularity, thus it is used for the derivation of the corrected score or log-likelihood function. In Augustin (2004) a corrected log-likelihood is considered, where in the Breslow log-likelihood X_i is replaced by A_i and the moment generating function is used for correction. In comparison to Augustin (2004) the corrected log-likelihood is extended for more than one error-prone variable. In addition, error-free covariables can be considered. Under the assumptions of the error model from Section 2.1.1 the corrected log-likelihood is given as follows

$$l_{corr}^A(\pi, A, \beta_X, h_j) = \sum_{j=1}^{k} \left[d_j ln(h_j) + \sum_{i \in D(\pi_j)} \beta_X' A_i - h_j(\pi_j - \pi_{j-1}) \sum_{i \in R(\pi_j)} \underbrace{\frac{exp(\beta_X' A_i)}{M_{U_i}(\beta_X)}}_{:=(*)} \right]$$

$$(2.24)$$

The correction for measurement error is only necessary for W_i. For the term (*) in Equation (2.24) this means in detail

$$(*) = \frac{exp\left((\beta_{V_1}, \cdots, \beta_{V_p}, \beta_{F_{p+1}}, \cdots, \beta_{F_m}) \cdot A_i\right)}{M_{U_i}(\beta_X)}$$

$$= \frac{exp\left(\beta_{V_1}W_{i1} + \ldots + \beta_{V_p}W_{ip} + \beta_{F_{p+1}}F_{ip+1} + \ldots + \beta_{F_m}F_{im}\right)}{M_{U_i}(\beta_X)}$$

$$\overset{U_i \perp \{V_i, F_i\}}{=} \frac{exp(\beta_{V_1}W_{i1})}{M_{U_i}(\beta_{V_1})} \cdot \ldots \cdot \frac{exp(\beta_{F_m}F_{im})}{M_{U_i}(\beta_{F_m})}$$

$$= exp(\beta_{V_1}W_{i1} - log[M_{U_i}(\beta_{V_1})]) \cdot \ldots \cdot exp(\beta_{F_m}F_{im} - log[M_{U_i}(\beta_{F_m})])$$

$$= exp(\beta_{V_1}W_{i1} - log[M_{U_i}(\beta_{V_1})] + \ldots + \beta_{F_m}F_{im} - \underbrace{log[M_{U_i}(\beta_{F_m})]}_{=1})$$

$$= exp(\beta_{V_1}W_{i1} - log[M_{U_i}(\beta_{V_1})] + \ldots + \beta_{V_p}W_{ip} - log[M_{U_i}(\beta_{V_p})] +$$
$$\beta_{F_{p+1}}F_{ip+1} + \ldots + \beta_{F_m}F_{im}).$$

The corresponding corrected score function $s^A_{corr_{\beta_X}}(\pi, A, \beta_X, h_j)$ is given by

$$\sum_{j=1}^{k} \left[\sum_{i \in D(\pi_j)} A_i - \frac{d_j}{\sum_{i \in R(\pi_j)} exp(\beta'_X A_i)/M_{U_i}(\beta_X)} \cdot \sum_{i \in R(\pi_j)} K_i(\beta_X, A_i, M_{U_i}) \right] = 0, \tag{2.25}$$

where $K_i(\beta_X, A_i, M_{U_i}) = exp(\beta'_X A_i)/M_{U_i}(\beta_X) \cdot \left(A_i - \frac{\partial}{\partial \beta_X} ln M_{U_i}(\beta_X)\right)$. The root of the corrected score function provides a corrected parameter estimation $\hat{\beta}^*_X$.
A corrected estimation of the cumulative baseline hazard $\hat{H}^*_0(t)$ is derived as

$$\hat{H}^*_0(t) = \sum_{j:\pi_j \leq t} \frac{d_j}{\sum_{i \in R(\pi_j)} exp(\beta'_X A_i)/M_{U_i}(\hat{\beta}^*_X)}. \tag{2.26}$$

The detailed calculations of $s^A_{corr_{\beta_X}}(\cdot)$ and $\hat{H}^*_0(t)$ are located in the Appendix B.2. It can be shown that the corrected log-likelihood satisfies condition (2.13) of being an unbiased estimation equation and accordingly the corrected score function fulfils the condition (2.12) with $\vartheta = (h_1, \ldots h_k, \beta_{V_1}, \cdots, \beta_{V_p}, \beta_{F_{p+1}}, \ldots, \beta_{F_m})$ and $\hat{Y} = (min(T_i, C_i), \delta_i)$, $i = 1, \ldots, n$. The proof is given in the Appendix B.1. In the case of normal homoscedastic errors $M_{U_i}(\beta) \equiv M_U(\beta)$ and is defined as

$$M_U(\beta_X) = exp\left(\frac{1}{2}\beta'_X \Sigma_U \beta_X\right), \tag{2.27}$$

with the m-dimensional vector $\beta_X = (\beta_{V_1}, \ldots, \beta_{V_p}, \beta_{F_{p+1}}, \ldots, \beta_{F_m})'$.

Inference on the parameter estimates

The resulting corrected parameter estimators are under certain regularity conditions consistent and asymptotically normal. For the inference on $\hat{\beta}_X^*$ M-estimation techniques are used (see Carroll et al., 2006, Chapter 7). The covariance matrix is derived via the *sandwich estimator* (also called *robust covariance estimator*):

$$Cov(\hat{\beta}_X^*) = I(\hat{\beta}_X^*)^{-1} C(\hat{\beta}_X^*) I(\hat{\beta}_X^*)^{-1}, \tag{2.28}$$

with the empirical observed (corrected) Fisher information matrix

$$I(\hat{\beta}_X^*) = -\frac{\partial s_{corr_{\hat{\beta}_X^*}}^A (\pi, A, \hat{\beta}_X^*, h_j)}{\partial \hat{\beta}_X^{*\prime}} \tag{2.29}$$

and matrix C, an estimate for the covariance matrix of the corrected score function,

$$C(\hat{\beta}_X^*) = \sum_{i=1}^n s_{corr_{\hat{\beta}_X^*}}^A (\pi, A, \hat{\beta}_X^*, h_j) s_{corr_{\hat{\beta}_X^*}}^A (\pi, A, \hat{\beta}_X^*, h_j)'. \tag{2.30}$$

The standard deviation is the root of the diagonal elements of the covariance matrix

$$se(\hat{\beta}_{X_J}^*) = \sqrt{Cov(\hat{\beta}_{X_J}^*)}_{[JJ]}, \tag{2.31}$$

with $J = 1, \ldots, m$ and m the number of covariates. An asymptotic $(1 - \alpha)\%$ confidence interval is defined by

$$\hat{\beta}_{X_J}^* \pm z_{1-\alpha/2} \cdot se(\hat{\beta}_{X_J}^*), \tag{2.32}$$

where $z_{1-\alpha/2}$ denotes the $(1 - \alpha/2)$-quantile of the standard normal distribution. To examine, if the individual covariable has an effect on the survival time, a Wald test with null hypothesis $H_0 : \beta_{X_J}^* = 0$ is conducted with test statistic

$$z = \frac{\hat{\beta}_{X_J}^*}{se(\hat{\beta}_{X_J}^*)}. \tag{2.33}$$

Under the null hypothesis z is standard normally distributed. The likelihood ratio test is used to check the significance of the entire model. The test compare the full model (with covariates) and the null model. The null hypothesis is

$H_0 : \beta^*_{X_1} = \ldots, \beta^*_{X_m} = 0$ and the test statistic is defined as follows:

$$LR = 2 \cdot (l^A_{corr}(\pi, A, \hat{\beta}^*_X, h_j) - l^0_{Br}), \tag{2.34}$$

where $l^A_{corr}(\cdot)$ is the corrected log-likelihood from Equation (2.24) evaluated at the corrected parameter estimates. For the null model no measurement error correction has to be conducted, because no covariable is considered, thus the Breslow likelihood evaluated at $X_i = 0$ (Equation (2.23)) is used denoted by l^0_{Br}. Under H_0 LR is χ^2 distributed with q degrees of freedom (q is the number of estimated parameters in the model).

Weibull Model

The concept of correction for measurement error can also be applied to some variants and generalizations of the Cox model (Augustin, 2004). Here, the Weibull model is considered.

The Weibull distribution in the Weibull model is parameterised as follows. Let $t \sim Wei(b, a)$ with density function

$$f(t) = b \cdot a \cdot (b \cdot t)^{a-1} \cdot exp(-(b \cdot t)^a), \tag{2.35}$$

where $b = exp(-\theta)$, $\theta = \beta'_X X$, $a = 1/\nu$ with $a, b, \nu > 0$ (Fahrmeir et al., 1996, Chapter 7). X_i and β_X are defined as in Equation (2.16) and (2.17). b denotes the scale parameter and $1/\nu$ the shape parameter of the Weibull distribution. From the distribution function $F(t) = 1 - exp(-(bt)^a)$ the survival function is derived, $S(t) = 1 - F(t) = exp(-(bt)^a)$. These results are used to specify the hazard rate and accordingly the baseline hazard rate:

$$h(t) = \frac{f(t)}{S(t)} = b \cdot a \cdot (b \cdot t)^{a-1} = b^a a \cdot t^{a-1} = \theta^* \cdot a \cdot t^{a-1} = \theta^* \cdot \frac{1}{\nu} \cdot t^{1/\nu-1} \tag{2.36}$$

$$h_0(t) = a \cdot t^{a-1} = \frac{1}{\nu} \cdot t^{1/\nu-1} \tag{2.37}$$

with $\theta^* = exp(-\theta a) = exp(-\theta/\nu)$. The cumulative hazard rate is derived as follows

$$H(t) = b^a \cdot a \int_0^t u^{a-1} du = b^a \cdot a \left[\frac{1}{a} u^a \right]_0^t = b^a t^a = b^{1/\nu} t^{1/\nu} \tag{2.38}$$

and thus

$$H_0(t) = t^a = t^{1/\nu}. \tag{2.39}$$

The model equation and the likelihood for the Weibull model can be set up in two different ways. In the following both versions are described.

Version 1

Motivated by the semi-parametric Cox model (see Equation (2.3)) the model equation for the Weibull model is defined as follows

$$h(t, X_i) = h_0(t) \cdot exp(X_i' \beta_X^+), \tag{2.40}$$

with $\beta_X^+ = -\beta_X/\nu$ and $h_0(t) = \frac{1}{\nu} \cdot t^{1/\nu-1}$ as derived in Equation (2.37). Substituting these results in the Breslow likelihood (see Equation (2.22)) leads to

$$L^X(\pi, X, \beta_X^+, \nu) = \prod_{i=1}^{n} \left[\left(\frac{1}{\nu} \cdot t_i^{1/\nu-1} \cdot exp(\beta_X^{+'} X_i) \right)^{\delta_i} exp\left(-exp(\beta_X^{+'} X_i) \cdot t_i^{1/\nu} \right) \right] \tag{2.41}$$

with $\int_0^{t_i} h_0(u)du = t^{1/\nu}$ (cumulative baseline hazard) and the log-likelihood is derived as follows:

$$l^X(\pi, X, \beta_X^+, \nu) = \sum_{i=1}^{n} \left[\delta_i \left(ln\left(\frac{1}{\nu} \cdot t_i^{1/\nu-1} \right) + \beta_X^{+'} X_i \right) - exp(\beta_X^{+'} X_i) \cdot t_i^{1/\nu} \right]. \tag{2.42}$$

A correction for ties is not considered, because in the Weibull model continuous failure times are assumed.

Version 2

The Weibull model for subject i, $i = 1, \ldots, n$, can also be written as a linear model for the logarithmic failure time T_i:

$$ln(T_i) = \beta_X' X_i + \nu \epsilon_i, \tag{2.43}$$

where ϵ_i is a random error, which has a standard extreme value distribution, $f(\epsilon_i) = exp(\epsilon_i)exp(-exp(\epsilon_i))$ (Fahrmeir et al., 1996, Chapter 7). The hazard rate and the survival function are given as follows:

$$h(y) = \frac{1}{\nu} exp\left(\frac{y - \theta}{\nu}\right) \tag{2.44}$$

$$S(y) = exp\left(-exp\left(\frac{y - \theta}{\nu}\right)\right) \tag{2.45}$$

with $y = ln(T)$ and $\theta = \beta'_X X$. The log-likelihood is defined by

$$l^X(\pi, X, \beta_X, \nu) = \sum_{i=1}^{n} [-\delta_i \cdot ln(\nu) + \delta_i log(h(y_i)) + log(S(y_i))] \tag{2.46}$$

$$= \sum_{i=1}^{n} \left[\delta_i \left[\left(\frac{y_i - \theta_i}{\nu}\right) - ln(\nu)\right] - exp\left(\frac{y_i - \theta_i}{\nu}\right)\right] \tag{2.47}$$

with $y_i = min(ln(T_i), ln(C_i))$ and $\theta_i = \beta'_X X_i$ (cf. Fahrmeir et al., 1996, Chapter 7). The details of transformation are located in Appendix B.3.1.

Equivalence of the two Versions

It is shown that the second version (Equation (2.47)) and first version (Equation (2.42) of the log-likelihood for the Weibull model are equivalent (see Appendix B.3.2). In the thesis it was decided for the second version, because this version is used in R package survival to fit a Weibull model via the survreg() function. In addition, instead of ν the logarithm of ν is considered in the survreg() function. This is useful for the inference on ν, which is done on the log scale to extend the range of ν from greater than zero to $(-\infty, +\infty)$. With $\tau = ln(\nu)$ and $\theta_i = \beta'_X X_i$ the log-likelihood from Equation (2.47) in given by

$$l^X(\pi, X, \beta_X, \nu) = \sum_{i=1}^{n} \left[\delta_i \left[\left(\frac{y_i - \beta'_X X_i}{exp(\tau)}\right) - \tau\right] - exp\left(\frac{y_i - \beta'_X X_i}{exp(\tau)}\right)\right]. \tag{2.48}$$

Corrected Log-Likelihood and Score Function of the Weibull Model

To make the results of the master's thesis comparable to those of the survreg() function the log-likelihood from Equation (2.48) is the base for the derivation of the corrected log-likelihood. According to Augustin (2004) the correction for measurement error is done via the moment generating function to allow for rather general types of error distributions. The corrected log-likelihood is derived as follows

$$l_{corr}^{A}(t, A, \beta_X, \tau) = \sum_{i=1}^{n} \left[\delta_i \left[\left(\frac{y_i - \beta_X' A_i}{exp(\tau)} \right) - \tau \right] - exp \left(\frac{y_i - \beta_X' A_i}{exp(\tau)} - ln(M_{U_i}(\beta_X^+)) \right) \right]$$

(2.49)

The corrected score functions are the derivatives with respect to β_X and τ and are given by

$$s_{corr_{\beta_X}}^{A}(t, A, \beta_X, \tau) = \sum_{i=1}^{n} \left[-\delta_i \left(\frac{A_i}{exp(\tau)} \right) + exp \left(\frac{y_i - \beta_X' A_i}{exp(\tau)} - ln(M_{U_i}(\beta_X^+)) \right) \cdot \right.$$
$$\left. \left(\frac{A_i}{exp(\tau)} + \frac{\partial}{\partial \beta_X} ln(M_{U_i}(\beta_X^+)) \right) \right],$$

(2.50)

$$s_{corr_{\tau}}^{A}(t, A, \beta_X, \tau) = \sum_{i=1}^{n} \left[-\delta_i \left[1 + \left(\frac{y_i - \beta_X' A_i}{exp(\tau)} \right) \right] + \right.$$
$$\left. exp \left(\frac{y_i - \beta_X' A_i}{exp(\tau)} - ln(M_{U_i}(\beta_X^+)) \right) \cdot \left[\frac{y_i - \beta_X' A_i}{exp(\tau)} + \frac{\partial}{\partial \tau} ln(M_{U_i}(\beta_X^+)) \right] \right].$$

(2.51)

The details of derivation are located in Appendix B.5. These corrected score functions are an extension to the suggested adjusted score functions for the Weibull model by Gimenez et al. (1999) from normal homoscedastic to non-normal heteroscedastic measurement errors. It can be shown that the corrected log-likelihood satisfies condition (2.13) of being an unbiased estimation equation and accordingly the corrected score functions fulfil the condition (2.12) with $\vartheta = (\beta_{V_1}, \cdots, \beta_{V_p}, \beta_{F_p+1}, \ldots, \beta_{F_m}, \tau)$ and $\tilde{Y} = (min(T_i, C_i), \delta_i)$, $i = 1, \ldots, n$. The proof is given in the Appendix B.4.

Corrected Log-Likelihood and Score Function for Homoscedatic Normal Measurement Errors

To specify the error model of Section 2.1.1, U_i is taken to be identically normally distributed with mean zero and known (or consistently estimated) covariance matrix Σ_U, $U_i \sim N(0, \Sigma_U)$, $i = 1, \ldots, n$. Thus, for the moment generating function

$M_{U_i}(\beta) \equiv M_U(\beta)$ holds and one obtains

$$M_U(\beta_X^+) = exp\left(\frac{1}{2}\beta_X^{+'}\Sigma_U\beta_X^+\right) \tag{2.52}$$

$$= exp\left(\frac{\beta_X'\Sigma_U\beta_X}{2 \cdot exp(\tau)^2}\right), \tag{2.53}$$

with the $(m+1)$-dimensional vector $\beta_X = (\beta_0, \beta_{V_1}, \ldots, \beta_{V_p}, \beta_{F_{p+1}}, \ldots, \beta_{F_m})'$. Furthermore,

$$ln(M_U(\beta_X^+)) = \frac{\beta_X'\Sigma_U\beta_X}{2 \cdot exp(\tau)^2} \tag{2.54}$$

$$\frac{\partial}{\partial\beta_X}lnM_U(\beta_X^+) = \frac{\beta_X\Sigma_U}{exp(\tau)^2} \tag{2.55}$$

$$\frac{\partial}{\partial\tau}lnM_U(\beta_X^+) = -\frac{\beta_X'\Sigma_U\beta_X}{exp(\tau)^2}. \tag{2.56}$$

A consistent estimator for $\hat{\Sigma}_U$ of Σ_U is assumed to exist. Usually, such estimators are derived using validation data (e.g. Kong and Gu (1999); Carroll et al. (2006, Chapter 3)). The adjustment for measurement error is only required for W_i. Thus the definition of $M_U(\beta_X)$ has to be extended to

$$M_U(\beta_X) = \begin{cases} exp\left(\frac{\beta_X'\Sigma_U\beta_X}{2 \cdot exp(\tau)^2}\right) & \text{if } W_J, \ J = 1, \ldots, p \\ 1 & \text{if } F_J, \ J = p+1, \ldots, m. \end{cases} \tag{2.57}$$

Substituting Equations (2.54) – (2.56) in (2.49), (2.50) and (2.51) leads to the corrected log-likelihood

$$l_{corr}^A(t, A, \beta_X, \tau) = \sum_{i=1}^{n}\left[\delta_i\left[\left(\frac{y_i - \beta_X'A_i}{exp(\tau)}\right) - \tau\right] - exp\left(\underbrace{\frac{y_i - \beta_X'A_i}{exp(\tau)} - \frac{\beta_X'\Sigma_U\beta_X}{2 \cdot exp(\tau)^2}}_{:=(\#)}\right)\right],$$

$$\tag{2.58}$$

to the corrected score function of β_X

$$s^A_{corr_{\beta_X}}(t, A, \beta_X, \tau) = \sum_{i=1}^{n} \left[-\delta_i \left(\frac{A_i}{exp(\tau)} \right) + exp \left(\frac{y_i - \beta'_X A_i}{exp(\tau)} - \frac{\beta'_X \Sigma_U \beta_X}{2 \cdot exp(\tau)^2} \right) \cdot \right.$$
$$\left. \left(\frac{A_i}{exp(\tau)} + \frac{\beta_X \Sigma_U}{exp(\tau)^2} \right) \right]$$
$$= \frac{1}{exp(\tau)} \sum_{i=1}^{n} \left[exp \left(\frac{y_i - \beta'_X A_i}{exp(\tau)} - \frac{\beta'_X \Sigma_U \beta_X}{2 \cdot exp(\tau)^2} \right) \cdot \left(A_i + \frac{\beta_X \Sigma_U}{exp(\tau)} \right) - \delta_i A_i \right],$$
$$(2.59)$$

and to the corrected score function of τ

$$s^A_{corr_\tau}(t, A, \beta_X, \tau)$$
$$= \sum_{i=1}^{n} \left[-\delta_i \left[1 + \left(\frac{y_i - \beta'_X A_i}{exp(\tau)} \right) \right] + exp \left(\frac{y_i - \beta'_X A_i}{exp(\tau)} - \frac{\beta'_X \Sigma_U \beta_X}{2 \cdot exp(\tau)^2} \right) \cdot \right.$$
$$\left. \left[\frac{y_i - \beta'_X A_i}{exp(\tau)} - \frac{\beta'_X \Sigma_U \beta_X}{exp(\tau)^2} \right] \right].$$
$$(2.60)$$

As mentioned above these equations correspond to the corrected log-likelihood and the corrected score functions under the assumption of normal homosecedastic measurement errors (cf. Gimenez et al., 1999).

The correction for measurement error is only necessary for W_i. For the term (#) in Equation (2.58) this means in detail

$$(\#) = \frac{y_i}{exp(\tau)} - \frac{\beta'_X A_i}{exp(\tau)} - \frac{\beta'_X \Sigma_U \beta_X}{2 \cdot exp(\tau)^2}$$
$$= \frac{y_i}{exp(\tau)} -$$
$$\left[\frac{\beta_0 + \beta_{V_1} W_{i1} + \ldots + \beta_{V_p} W_{ip} + \beta_{F_{p+1}} F_{ip+1} + \ldots + \beta_{F_m} F_{im}}{exp(\tau)} + \frac{\beta'_X \Sigma_U \beta_X}{2 \cdot exp(\tau)^2} \right]$$
$$\stackrel{U_i \perp \{V_i, F_i\}}{=} \frac{y_i}{exp(\tau)} - \left[\frac{\beta_0}{exp(\tau)} + \frac{\beta_{V_1} W_{i1}}{exp(\tau)} + \frac{\beta_{V_1}^2 \sigma^2_{U_{V_1}}}{2 \cdot exp(\tau)^2} + \ldots + \frac{\beta_{V_p} W_{ip}}{exp(\tau)} + \frac{\beta_{V_p}^2 \sigma^2_{U_{V_p}}}{2 \cdot exp(\tau)^2} \right.$$
$$\left. + \ldots + \frac{\beta_{F_{p+1}} F_{ip+1}}{exp(\tau)} + \frac{\beta_{F_{p+1}}^2 \sigma^2_{U_{F_{p+1}}}}{2 \cdot exp(\tau)^2} + \ldots + \frac{\beta_{F_m} F_{im}}{exp(\tau)} + \frac{\beta_{F_m}^2 \sigma^2_{U_{F_m}}}{2 \cdot exp(\tau)^2} \right]$$

$$
\overset{2.57}{=} \frac{y_i}{exp(\tau)} - \left[\frac{\beta_0}{exp(\tau)} + \frac{\beta_{V_1} W_{i1}}{exp(\tau)} + \frac{\beta_{V_1}^2 \sigma_{U_{V_1}}^2}{2 \cdot exp(\tau)^2} + \ldots + \frac{\beta_{V_p} W_{ip}}{exp(\tau)} + \frac{\beta_{V_p}^2 \sigma_{U_{V_p}}^2}{2 \cdot exp(\tau)^2} \right.
$$
$$
\left. + \ldots + \frac{\beta_{F_{p+1}} F_{ip+1}}{exp(\tau)} + \ldots + \frac{\beta_{F_m} F_{im}}{exp(\tau)} \right].
$$

The roots of the corrected score functions are the corrected parameter estimators $\hat{\beta}_X^*$ and $\hat{\tau}^*$.

Inference on the parameter estimates

The calculation of the standard deviation for the corrected parameter estimators as well as the Wald and likelihood ratio test are computed in the same way as for the Cox model. The covariance matrix for $\hat{\vartheta}^* = \left(\hat{\beta}_X^*, \hat{\tau}^* \right)$ with

$$
s_{corr_{\hat{\vartheta}^*}}^A = \left(s_{corr_{\hat{\beta}_X^*}}^A (t, A, \hat{\beta}_X^*, \hat{\tau}^*), s_{corr_{\hat{\tau}^*}}^A (t, A, \hat{\beta}_X^*, \hat{\tau}^*) \right)' \tag{2.61}
$$

are derived via the *sandwich estimator*:

$$
Cov(\hat{\vartheta}^*) = I(\hat{\vartheta}^*)^{-1} C(\hat{\vartheta}^*) I(\hat{\vartheta}^*)^{-1} \tag{2.62}
$$

with the empirical observed (corrected) Fisher information matrix

$$
I(\hat{\vartheta}^*) = -\frac{\partial s_{corr_{\hat{\vartheta}^*}}^A (\pi, A, \hat{\vartheta}^*)}{\partial \hat{\vartheta}^*} = - \begin{pmatrix} \frac{\partial s_{corr_{\hat{\beta}_X^*}}^A (t, A, \hat{\beta}_X^*, \hat{\tau}^*)}{\partial \hat{\beta}_X^*} & \frac{\partial s_{corr_{\hat{\beta}_X^*}}^A (t, A, \hat{\beta}_X^*, \hat{\tau}^*)}{\partial \hat{\tau}^*} \\ \frac{\partial s_{corr_{\hat{\tau}^*}}^A (t, A, \hat{\beta}_X^*, \hat{\tau}^*)}{\partial \hat{\beta}_X^*} & \frac{\partial s_{corr_{\hat{\tau}^*}}^A (t, A, \hat{\beta}_X^*, \hat{\tau}^*)}{\partial \hat{\tau}^*} \end{pmatrix} \tag{2.63}
$$

and matrix C

$$
C(\hat{\vartheta}^*) = \sum_{i=1}^n s_{corr_{\hat{\vartheta}^*}}^A (\pi, A, \hat{\vartheta}^*) \, s_{corr_{\hat{\vartheta}^*}}^A (\pi, A, \hat{\vartheta}^*)'. \tag{2.64}
$$

The standard deviation is the root of the diagonal elements of the covariance matrix

$$
se(\hat{\beta}_{X_J}^*) = \sqrt{Cov(\hat{\vartheta}^*)}_{[JJ]}, \tag{2.65}
$$

where $J = 1, \ldots, m$ with m the number of covariates and

$$
se(\hat{\tau}^*) = \sqrt{Cov(\hat{\vartheta}^*)}_{[qq]}, \tag{2.66}
$$

with q is the number of estimated parameters. A $(1 - \alpha)\%$ asymptotic confidence interval for $\hat{\beta}_X^*$ and $\hat{\tau}^*$ is defined by

$$\hat{\beta}_{X_J}^* \pm z_{1-\alpha/2} \cdot se(\hat{\beta}_{X_J}^*) \tag{2.67}$$

and

$$\hat{\tau}^* \pm z_{1-\alpha/2} \cdot se(\hat{\tau}^*), \tag{2.68}$$

where $z_{1-\alpha/2}$ is the $(1 - \alpha/2)$-quantile of the standard normal distribution. The confidence interval for $\hat{v}^* = exp(\hat{\tau}^*)$ (this holds because of the invariance of maximum-likelihood estimator) is yielded by taking the exponential function of the lower and upper boundary of the confidence interval for $\hat{\tau}^*$.

To examine, if the individual parameter estimators have a significant effect, a Wald test with null hypothesis $H_0 : \beta_{X_J}^* = 0$ and $H_0 : \tau^* = 0$, respectively, is conducted with test statistic

$$z = \frac{\hat{\beta}_{X_J}^*}{se(\hat{\beta}_{X_J}^*)} \overset{H_0}{\sim} N(0,1) \tag{2.69}$$

and

$$z = \frac{\hat{\tau}^*}{se(\hat{\tau}^*)} \overset{H_0}{\sim} N(0,1). \tag{2.70}$$

The likelihood ratio test is used to check the significance of the entire model. The null hypothesis is $H_0 : \beta_{X_1}^* = \ldots, \beta_{X_m}^* = \tau^* = 0$ and the test statistic is defined as follows:

$$LR = 2 \cdot (l_{corr}^A(\pi, A, \hat{\vartheta}^*) - l_0^X) \overset{H_0}{\sim} \chi^2(q), \tag{2.71}$$

where $l_{corr}^A(\cdot)$ is the corrected log-likelihood from Equation (2.49) or (2.58) evaluated at the corrected parameter estimates and l_0^X is uncorrected log-likelihood from Equation (2.48) evaluated at $X_i = 0$.

2.2. Model-Based Recursive Partitioning

In this thesis an adjustment for measurement errors in Cox and Weibull models is incorporated in the framework of model-based recursive partitioning, which was developed by Zeileis et al. (2008). Therefore, the described corrected log-likelihoods and corrected score functions are integrated into the algorithm of model-based recursive partitioning that relies on score functions. Model-based recursive partitioning is related to the method of classification and regression trees, which is outlined in the next section.

2.2.1. Introduction to Classification and Regression Trees

The basic idea of *classification and regression trees* (CART) is to split successively the feature space of the covariates into subsets that have similar response values within each other, but different values between each other (Fahrmeir et al., 1996, Chapter 5). These methods have their origin in the so-called automatic interaction detection (AID), which was derived by Morgan and Sonquist (1963).

From a statistical point of view the algorithm of classification and regression trees underlies the global hypothesis that the covariates are <u>not</u> related to the response variable. Starting with the whole sample, the global hypothesis is tested. If the null hypothesis cannot be rejected, the algorithm stops, otherwise the covariable with the largest association is chosen for splitting. Thereby, different criteria for the selection of the splitting variable are employed. For example entropy measures such as the Gini Index and Shannon Entropy are used (cf. Strobl et al., 2009). In modern classification tree algorithm association tests with related p-values, where the variable with the minimal p-value is chosen for partitioning, are used (cf. Hothorn et al., 2006). In the next step, an optimal split point for the selected splitting variable has to be determined, so that the discrepancy in the response variable between the subgroups is maximal. The cut point is used to split the sample into subgroups according to the selected covariate. These two steps are repeated until no more significant association is detected. Successively, a tree structure develops, which is characterised by its nodes. A node consists of the subset of the feature space, which should be split in the next step. If the response variable is categorical, the tree is called *classification tree* and if it is continuous, the tree is called *regression tree*. Because of the successive partitioning, which is based on the step before, this procedure is also named as *recursive partitioning*.

An example for a tree is given in Figure 2.1. The Lung Cancer Data, which is available in the R package survival (Therneau and Lumley, 2009), includes the censored survival data for patients with advanced lung cancer. The survival time (in days) is split with respect to *ph.ecog*, which describes the ECOG performance score (0 = good, 5 = dead), into groups less or equal than 1 and greater than 1. The group with a good ECOG performance score is partitioned further for *sex* (male = 1, female = 2). The tree structure shows an interaction effect between *ph.ecog* and *sex*. In the terminal nodes the estimated survival curves for the resulting subsets

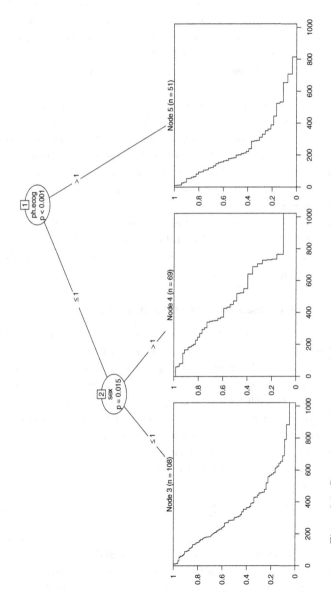

Figure 2.1.: Recursive partitioning with Lung Cancer Data, generated in R with the function ctree ()

are shown. The advantages of this approach are that they are also applicable, if the number of predictor variables is greater than the number of observations, e. g. in gene expression data (Strobl et al., 2009). In addition, interactions are automatically detected. The most popular algorithm for classification and regression trees are CART and C4.5, which were derived by Breiman et al. (1984) and independently by Quinlan (1986).

Fundamental problems of classification and regression trees are variable selection bias and overfitting. A classic strategy to deal with overfitting is to *prune* the trees after growing them (Strobl et al., 2009). Hothorn et al. (2006) suggest an algorithm for binary recursive partitioning, which uses the p-values of a permutation test for variable selection and for finding the optimal split point. The p-values and a minimal sample size per node operate as a stopping criterion, thus the trees do not depend on pruning.

Extensions of the single classification trees are *bagging* (Breiman, 1996, 1998) and *random forest* (Breiman, 2001). They belong to the so-called *ensemble methods*, which use averages over a sample of trees. The advantage of these methods is a better prediction, but worse interpretability.

2.2.2. Model-Based Recursive Partitioning

A variant of recursive partitioning is model-based recursive partitioning (MOB), which was derived by Zeileis et al. (2008). MOB is a combination of non-parametric classification trees and parametric models and is therefore a semi-parametric approach. In comparison to classification and regression trees, MOB does not aim to find subsets with different values of the response variable, but with different values of the model parameters. By partitioning the data with regard to certain covariates a better conformation of the model to the data should be achieved.

Let $Y_i, i = 1, \ldots, n$, be the dependent variable and ϑ be a q-dimensional vector of model parameters. The model parameters are estimated by minimizing a certain objective function $\Psi(Y, \vartheta)$

$$\sum_{i=1}^{n} \Psi(Y_i, \vartheta) \rightarrow min. \qquad (2.72)$$

For example in generalized linear regression models for the maximum likelihood estimation, $\Psi(\cdot)$ is replaced by the negative log-likelihood.

In some situations it is inadequate to fit one global model for the given data set. By partitioning the data with respect to so-called *partitioning variables* $Z_j, j = 1, \ldots, l$, a better model fit should be achieved. In the following the steps of model-based recursive partitioning are outlined (Zeileis et al., 2008):

Given are $X_1, \ldots, X_m$ independent variables and $Z_1, \ldots, Z_l$ partitioning variables. $Y_1 \ldots, Y_n$ describe the values of the dependent variable.

1. The model is estimated with all observations in the current node. Thereby, the parameter estimators $\hat{\vartheta}$ are obtained by minimizing $\Psi(Y_i, \vartheta)$.

2. Conduct a test for parameter instability to assess whether the parameter estimation related to the partitioning variables $Z_1, \ldots, Z_l$ is stable. If there is some overall instability, select the variable Z_j^* with the highest parameter instability. Otherwise stop the algorithm.

3. Compute the cut point ξ for the partitioning variable Z_j^*, which locally optimizes $\Psi(Y_i, \vartheta)$.

4. Split the nodes into daughter nodes with respect to the cut point ξ from step 3 and repeat the procedure from step 2.

The algorithm is conducted as long as in the second step no (more) significant parameter instability occurs, such that each node in the tree is related to a parametric model. The objective function $\Psi(Y_i, \vartheta)$ is used to judge the parameter instability in step 2 and to compute the cut points in step 3.

An example of a regression tree, which is computed by the MOB algorithm, is depicted in Figure 2.2. This example is taken from Zeileis et al. (2008). For the Pima Indians diabetes data (which is available in the R package mlbench (Leisch and Dimitriadou, 2010)) with n = 724 Pima Indian women and binary response variable positive/negative diabetes test, a MOB is computed based on a logistic regression. The plasma glucose concentration is included as a regressor. Five prognostic variables are considered as partitioning variables. A minimal subsample size of 20 and a significance level of 5% is chosen. As shown in Figure 2.2 the data is first split by a body mass index (*mass*) of 26.3. Those observations, which are in the group of higher body mass index, are further partitioned with respect to age in groups of under and over 30 years, respectively. The tree structure shows an interaction effect between *mass* and *age*. In the terminal nodes the response variable *diabetes*, a binary variable, and the covariate *glucose*, a numeric variable, are visualized in a spinogram.

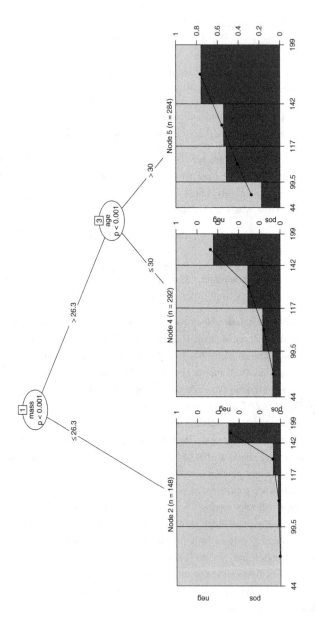

Figure 2.2.: MOB with Pima Indians data, generated in R with the function mob()

The idea of MOB in the generalized linear model (here logistic regression) in the example above can also be applied to other parametric regression models without further modification (Zeileis et al., 2008). Here, the Cox and Weibull model is considered to model censored survival data. In this thesis a correction for measurement error should be incorporated into the MOB algorithm. For the objective function $\Psi(Y_i, \vartheta)$, the corrected log-likelihood for the Cox and Weibull model, which were derived in Section 2.1.3, are adopted. This is possible, because the corrected score functions of the Cox and Weibull model fulfil the condition of being an unbiased estimation equation, this corresponds to the corrected score functions have zero expectation at the true parameters (see Appendix B.1 and B.4).

In detail step 1–3 of the MOB algorithm is described in the following. Additionally, the application to the Cox and Weibull model with correction for measurement error will be integrated into the algorithm. To simplify the notation, the dependence on the current node is omitted. In the following n is the number of observations in the current node. $\hat{\vartheta}$ stands for the parameter estimate in the according fitted model and B is the number of daughter nodes.

Step 1: Parameter Estimation

The model is fitted by minimizing the objective function $\Psi(Y_i, \vartheta)$. To adjust for measurement error the negative corrected log-likelihood has to be considered, which is denoted by $\Psi_{corr}(Y_i, \vartheta)$ in the following. The root of the corrected score function provide the corrected parameter estimator $\hat{\vartheta}^*$

$$\sum_{i=1}^{n} \psi_{corr}(Y_i, \hat{\vartheta}^*) = 0, \tag{2.73}$$

where

$$\psi_{corr}(Y_i, \hat{\vartheta}) = \frac{\partial}{\partial \vartheta} \Psi_{corr}(Y_i, \vartheta).$$

In the case of fitting the Cox model with $\vartheta = (h_1, \ldots, h_k, \beta_X)$ the negative corrected log-likelihood is given by $\Psi_{corr}(Y_i, \vartheta) = -l_{corr}^A(t, A, \beta_X, h_j)$ (see Equation (2.24)) and the negative corrected score function $\psi_{corr}(Y_i, \vartheta) = -(s_{corr_{\beta_X}}^A(t, A, \beta_X, h_j), s_{corr_{h_j}}^A(t, A, \beta_X, h_j))$ from Equation (2.25) and Appendix B.2. Accordingly, for fitting a corrected Weibull model, with $\vartheta = (\beta_X, \tau)$, $\Psi_{corr}(Y_i, \vartheta) = -l_{corr}^A(t, A, \beta_X, \tau)$ from Equation (2.58) and $\psi_{corr}(Y_i, \vartheta) = -(s_{corr_{\beta_X}}^A(t, A, \beta_X, \tau), s_{corr_{\tau}}^A(t, A, \beta_X, \tau))$ from Equation (2.59) and (2.60). In both models, the optimization of the log-likelihood is conducted iteratively.

To simplify matters in the following the negative corrected log-likelihood and the negative corrected score function for the Cox and Weibull model are only named by $\Psi_{corr}(\cdot)$ and $\psi_{corr}(\cdot)$.

Step 2: Test for Parameter Instability

Parameter instability in a parametric model can be described by structural change. A parameter instability is given, if the observations with respect to a certain ordering show a structural change, however, the breakpoint is unknown (Zeileis and Hornik, 2007). A score-based fluctuation test is conducted for parameter instability to assess whether the partitioning in the current node is necessary.

The null hypothesis, the parameter stability is satisfied,

$$H_0^j : \vartheta_{(i)} = \vartheta_0 \ (i = 1, \ldots, n; j = 1, \ldots, l) \tag{2.74}$$

is tested against the alternative that at least one component of $\vartheta_{(i)}$ varies over Z_j, where the index (i) denotes an ordering with respect to Z_j. If the global null hypothesis $H_0 = \bigcap_{j=1}^{l} H_0^j$ is rejected for a specified significance level α, the partitioning variable Z_j with the smallest p-value is selected with the intention to improve the model fit.

The idea of the test is to assess whether the model scores $\hat{\psi}_i = \psi(Y_i, \hat{\vartheta})$ fluctuate randomly around its mean 0. Thus, for the underlying score function the condition $E[\psi(Y, \vartheta_0)] = 0$ has to be hold, where ϑ_0 is the true parameter. For the Cox and Weibull model the corrected score function $\psi_{corr}(\cdot)$ fulfils the condition $E[\psi_{corr}(Y_i, \vartheta_0)] = 0$, see Appendix B.1 and B.4. If a systematic deviation from 0 over Z_j is observed, a parameter instability with respect to Z_j can be assumed.

To assess the parameter instability in the current node a *M-fluctuation test* is conducted, which was established by Zeileis and Hornik (2007). The M-fluctuation tests are always derived by the following steps (Zeileis and Hornik, 2007):

1. An appropriate estimation technique has to be chosen, e. g. the score function to fit the model, which satisfies the condition $E[\psi(Y, \vartheta_0)] = 0$.

2. An *empirical partial sum process* is used to capture the instabilities in the estimated model, which is governed by a *functional central limit theorem*.

3. The fluctuation within this process is measured by a *scalar functional*, which

is used to construct a test statistic. The test statistic is compared with the distribution of the limiting process.

In the case of the Cox and Weibull model with measurement error the procedure is as follows: Assuming H_0 is true, the corrected parameter estimate $\hat{\vartheta}^*$ is computed once for the full sample. The corrected estimator $\hat{\vartheta}^*$ is used to compute $\hat{\psi}_{corr} = \psi_{corr}(Y_i, \hat{\vartheta}^*)$. Under the alternative, we expect systematic deviation from the mean 0. The deviation is captured by the *empirical fluctuation process*, which is given by

$$W_j(t) = \hat{J}^{-1/2} n^{-1/2} \sum_{i=1}^{\lfloor nt \rfloor} \hat{\psi}_{corr_{\sigma(Z_{ij})}} \quad (0 \leq t \leq 1), \tag{2.75}$$

where $\sigma(Z_{ij})$ is the i-th ordered observation with respect to the j-th partitioning variable $Z_j = (Z_{1j}, \ldots, Z_{nj})'$ and $\lfloor \cdot \rfloor$ denotes the integer part of nt with $t \in [0, 1]$. $W_j(t)$ is the empirical partial sum score process ordered by the variable Z_j and scaled by the number of observations n and a consistent and non-singular estimate $\hat{J}$ of the covariance matrix $cov(\hat{\psi}_{corr}(Y, \hat{\vartheta}))$. Here, the covariance matrix is estimated by $\hat{J} = n^{-1} \sum_{i=1}^{n} \hat{\psi}_{corr}(Y_i, \hat{\vartheta}^*) \hat{\psi}_{corr}(Y_i, \hat{\vartheta}^*)'$.

Under the null hypothesis the empirical fluctuation process $W_j(t)$ follows the functional central limit theorem. This means that $W_j(t)$ converges to a Brownian bridge $W^0 = W(t) - tW(1)$ (Zeileis and Hornik, 2007).

A scalar functional $\lambda(\cdot)$ is used to construct a test statistic, which captures the empirical fluctuation process. For $\lambda(W_j(t))$ the functional limit theorem is also applied, thus the limiting process is $\lambda(W^0(t))$.

Zeileis (2005) gives an overview of three classes of structural change tests. The three classes are ML scores (Nyblom, 1989; Hansen, 1992; Hjort and Koning, 2002), F statistics including Wald, LR and LM test statistics (Andrews, 1993; Andrews and Ploberger, 1994) as well as fluctuation tests based on OLS residuals CUSUM (Ploberger and Krämer, 1992) and MOSUM (Chu et al., 1995). They are embedded in the framework of generalized M-fluctuation tests. Any of these tests can be applied for detecting parameter instability in the MOB algorithm. Zeileis et al. (2008) suggest two test statistics for continuous and categorical partitioning variables Z_j, respectively, which are based on the class of F statistics.

To assess the parameter instability over a <u>numerical variable</u> Z_j, the test statistic is given as follows

$$\lambda_{supLM}(W_j) = \max_{i=\underline{i}, \ldots, \bar{i}} \left(\frac{i}{n} \cdot \frac{n-1}{n} \right)^{-1} \left\| W_j \left(\frac{i}{n} \right) \right\|_2^2, \tag{2.76}$$

with $\left\| W_j \left(\frac{i}{n} \right) \right\|_2^2 = W_j \left(\frac{i}{n} \right)' W_j \left(\frac{i}{n} \right)$. If $W_j(t)$ is considered as a function of the fraction of the sample size $1/n$, under the null hypothesis the path of $W_j(t)$ corresponds to a random process with constant zero mean (see also Strobl et al., 2010). The correction for measurement error in the test statistic is integrated over $W_j(\cdot)$ as defined in Equation (2.75). $\lambda_{supLM}(W_j)$ denotes the maximum of the squared L_2 norm of the empirical fluctuation process $W_j(\cdot)$ and is scaled by its variance function. The potential breakpoint is shifted over the interval $[\underline{i}, \bar{i}]$, where $\underline{i}$ is some minimal segment size and $\bar{i} = n - \underline{i}$. $\lambda_{supLM}(W_j)$ converges to the supremum of a tied-down Bessel process $sup_t(t(1-t))^{-1} \| W^0(t) \|_2^2$ from which the corresponding p-value p_j are computed (Zeileis et al., 2008).

To assess the parameter instability over a categorical variable Z_j with C different categories, the test statistic is given as follows

$$\lambda_{\chi^2}(W_j) = \sum_{c=1}^{C} \frac{|I_c|^{-1}}{n} \left\| \Delta_{I_c} W_j \left(\frac{i}{n} \right) \right\|_2^2 . \tag{2.77}$$

The test statistic is different in comparison to numerical partitioning variables, because Z_j has ties, therefore a total ordering of the observations is not possible. $\Delta_{I_c} W_j$ denotes the increment of the empirical fluctuation process over the observations in category $c = 1, \ldots, C$ and I_c is the sum of scores in category c. $\lambda_{\chi^2}(W_j)$ is the weighted sum of the squared L_2 norm of the increments. The test statistic is asymptotically χ^2-distributed with $q \cdot (C-1)$ degrees of freedom from which the corresponding p-value p_j are computed, where q is number of estimated parameters. In summary the steps for the derivation of the M-fluctuation test in the case of the Cox and Weibull model are as follows:

1. As an estimation technique the corrected score functions $\psi_{corr}(\cdot)$ for the Cox and Weibull model are chosen, which fulfil the condition of unbiased estimation by their definition (see Appendix B.1 and B.4 for the proof).

2. The *empirical partial sum process* $W_j(t)$ is used to capture the instabilities in the estimated model as defined in Equation (2.75) including the corrected score function. Under the null hypothesis $W_j(t)$ converges to a Brownian bridge.

3. A *scalar functional* $\lambda(\cdot)$ is used to construct a test statistic, which is based on the class of F statistics. The test statistic for continuous and categorical partitioning variables is defined in Equation (2.76) and (2.77), respectively.

The correction for measurement error is considered via $W_j(\cdot)$ from step 2.

The advantage of this approach is that the parameter estimates and the corresponding score functions only have to be computed once in a node (Zeileis et al., 2008), because the individual deviation is the same, only the ordering and the corresponding path of $W_j(t)$ has to be modified for computing the test statistics for the different partitioning variables. This means that for the empirical fluctuation process in Equation (2.75) the scores only have to be reordered for the different partitioning variables and be involved in the test statistic from Equation (2.76) and (2.77), respectively.

For each partitioning variable Z_j, $j = 1, \ldots, l$, the test statistic $\lambda(W_j)$ with associated p-values p_j is computed. The overall instability in the current node is assessed by checking whether the minimal p-value $\min_{j=1,\ldots,l} p_j$ falls below a pre-specified significance level α. The larger the number of partitioning variables is, the higher the false-positive rate is. To account for this problem of multiple testing a Bonferroni adjustment for the p-value is applied. Moreover, the test procedure in the tree is recursively nested. A significant p-value is only interpretable if the overall parameter instability has been rejected in all previous nodes in the tree. Thus, the recursive partitioning approach forms a closed test procedure and the specified significance level α holds for the entire tree (Strobl et al., 2010). The variable Z_{j*} with the minimal p-value is chosen for splitting the model in the next step of the algorithm.

Step 3: Split into Nodes

The fitted model should be split for a partitioning variable Z_{j*} into a segmented model with B segments. In the following, binary splitting is assumed, this means that $B = 2$. For computing multi-way splits, see Zeileis et al. (2008). The optimal cut point ξ for Z_{j*} is computed by maximizing the partitioned corrected log-likelihood over all candidate cut points. For a metric splitting variable, let $L(\xi) = (i|Z_{ij} \leq \xi)$ be the subsample before and $R(\xi) = (i|Z_{ij} > \xi)$ be the subsample after the cut point ξ. For both subsamples, the corrected parameter estimators $\hat{\vartheta}^{(L)*}$ and $\hat{\vartheta}^{(R)*}$ are computed by optimizing the corrected log-likelihood $\Psi_{corr}(Y_i, \vartheta)$. The partitioned corrected log-likelihood, given by the sum of the corrected log-likelihoods for the observations before and after the cut point ξ, is defined as follows

$$\sum_{i\in L(\xi)} \Psi_{corr}\left(Y_i, \hat{\vartheta}^{(L)*}\right) + \sum_{i\in R(\xi)} \Psi_{corr}\left(Y_i, \hat{\vartheta}^{(R)*}\right) \tag{2.78}$$

and is minimized over all candidate cut points ξ (Strobl et al., 2010). For categorical splitting variables the number of splits cannot be greater than the number of categories in the variable ($B \leq C$). In the case of binary splitting, a nominal partitioning variable can be split into any two groups. The one with the minimal partitioned corrected log-likelihood is chosen. In the case of a binary partitioning variable the cut point is trivial.

Step 2-4 are conducted recursively until a stopping criterion is reached. Two kinds of stopping criteria are embedded in the MOB algorithm (Strobl et al., 2010):

1. If no (more) significant parameter instability for any partitioning variable Z_j is detected in step 2, the splitting stops. This means that the global null hypothesis cannot be rejected at a significance level α. Thus, the significance level α describes an important stopping criterion.

2. For step 3 a minimal sample size per node can be specified. The algorithm stops as soon as the minimal sample size per node is reached. The value of the minimal split size should be chosen, so that it provides a sufficient basis for parameter estimation in each subsample. The minimal sample size should be increased, if the number of parameters to be estimated is large.

In the following a few practical issues as well as pros and cons of the model-based recursive partitioning are outlined. The significance level and the minimal subsample size have to be specified by the researcher in advance. Commonly the significance level is 5%. Lower values should be chosen, if the sample size and/or the number of covariates are large, to avoid overfitting (Strobl et al., 2010).

Before the regression model is partitioned, the researcher has to decide, if a certain variable is included in the algorithm as a regressor or as a partitioning variable. This decision usually is based on the researcher's previous knowledge. For example, in biometric surveys a dose-response relationship would be fitted and partitioned with respect to further experiment-specific covariates (Zeileis et al., 2008).

An advantage of the model-based recursive partitioning is that the tree-structured regression analysis is easy to interpret by visualizing the fitted tree graphically. In addition, an automated variable selection is included, which is controlled for the Type I error rate in each node (cf. Kopf et al., 2010).

A problem in regression trees is overfitting or a selection bias with many possible splits (Hothorn et al., 2006). In the MOB algorithm variable selection bias is overcome by constructing a closed test procedure, which is controlled by α and by a separated variable and split point selection.

Another problem of recursive partitioning is the so-called *XOR-problem*. This problem occurs, if two covariates show no main effect, but a perfect interaction (Strobl et al., 2009). If none of the two covariates is selected in the first split of a classification tree, the interaction will never be detected. To overcome this problem, in the MOB algorithm interaction terms can be added to the list of partitioning variables (Zeileis et al., 2008).

3. Implementation

In Section 2.2.2 the integration of the Cox and Weibull model with adjustment for measurement error into the MOB algorithm is derived theoretically. For the implementation the focus is set to the Weibull model. In the R package `party` (Hothorn et al., 2010) a function `mob()` (Zeileis et al., 2008) is available to conduct model-based recursive partitioning. A detailed vignette for `mob()` is available in Zeileis et al. (2010). A model-based parameter estimation is already integrated for the Weibull model. The main challenge of the thesis is to extend the implemented estimation for the Weibull model with measurement error correction. For the implementation R version 2.11.1 (R Development Core Team, 2010) is used. The functionality of `mob()` and the extended implementation are described in the following.

3.1. Model-Based Recursive Partitioning in R

The default function call of `mob()` is

```
mob(formula, weights, data = list(), na.action = na.omit,
  model = glinearModel, control = mob_control(), ...)
```

The following information are taken from ?mob. The model `formula` to be fit is of type y ~ x1 + ... + xk | z1 + ... + zl, where the variables before | are considered in the model as covariables and the variables after | as partitioning variables. In `weights` a vector of non-negative weights can be specified, which is used in the fitting algorithm. This argument is optional and by default equal to 1. A `data` frame has to be passed containing the variables specified in the model `formula`. The handling of missing values is defined in `na.action`. The default is `na.omit`, in the case of a missing value the whole row is removed from the data frame. This means that the fitted model only is based on complete cases. In `model` the class of the model to be fit is specified and has to be of class `StatModel`. This class is provided by the package modeltools (Hothorn et al., 2010). This package is automatically loaded with party. Three StatModel objects are already available in modeltools. linearModel and glinearModel fit a (generalized) linear regression model, survReg fits a Weibull model. By default a glinearModel is fitted. New user-defined objects can be created by new('StatModel', ...).

control contains a list of control parameters for the MOB algorithm and is returned by mob_control():

```
mob_control(alpha = 0.05, bonferroni = TRUE, minsplit = 20,
   trim = 0.1, objfun = deviance, breakties = FALSE,
   parm = NULL, verbose = FALSE)
```

By default the significance level alpha for the parameter instability test is set to 0.05. The overall instability in the current node is assessed by checking whether any (possibly Bonferroni-corrected) p-value falls below alpha. By default bonferroni-corrected p-values are used in the parameter instability test. If bonferroni is set to FALSE the unadjusted p-values are considered. The minimal sample size per node is denoted by minsplit and by default equal to 20. Thus the two kinds of stopping criteria in the MOB algorithm, the significance level alpha and the minimal sample size minsplit, as described in Section 2.2.2, can be varied in mob_control(). Furthermore, the trimming parameter (trim) in the parameter instability test for numerical partitioning variables can be varied. By default it is set to 0.1. If the value is smaller than 1, it is interpreted as the fraction relative to the current node size. The function objfun extracts the value of the objective function from a fitted model in the current node and is used in step 3 of the MOB algorithm to find the optimal cut point. By default the deviance is extracted. breakties is of type logical. If breakties = TRUE, ties of numerical variables are broken randomly for computing the test statistics of parameter instability. By default it is set to FALSE. The number or name of model parameters that should be included in the test of parameter instability is specified by parm. By default all parameters are included. If the logical argument verbose is set to TRUE the details of the fitting process are printed on the R console. This includes the results of the parameter instability test (test statistics and p-values) and the selected splitting variables with their cut points.

In addition, further arguments can be passed to the function mob(,...). For example, to fit a glinearModel the family could be specified. By default family is equal to gaussian. In the case of a binomial model an additional argument would be `family = binomial()`.

In the following the procedure of the function `mob()` is embedded in the steps of the model-based recursive partitioning as described in Section 2.2.2:

Given are x1,...,xm independent variables and z1,...,zl partitioning variables. The values of the dependent variable are described by y. At first, the model `formula = y ~ x1 + ... + xk | z1 + ... + zl` and the data are prepared by the function `dpp()` (data preprocessing) for the MOB algorithm.

Step 1: Parameter estimation

The `model` with the specified `formula` is optimized with all observations in the current node via a `fit` function. For example, in the case of `linearModel` the fit function is equal to `lm.fit`, the usual function to fit a linear model in R. In the case of `survReg` the model is fitted via `survreg` with `dist = 'weibull'` (default), the usual function to fit a Weibull model in R.

Step 2: Test for Parameter Instability

A test for parameter instability is conducted to assess whether the parameter estimation related to the partitioning variables z1,...,zl is stable. To perform the parameter instability fluctuation test, a function `weights()` and a function `estfun()` is needed. The `weights()` function extracts the weights of an object of class `model` to determine which observations are in the current node. The observations in the node have weights greater than zero and those ones, which are not in the node, have weights equal to zero. `estfun()` returns a $(n \times q)$-matrix containing the values of the empirical estimating function for each observation. The estimating function for a model is the derivative of the objective function with respect to the parameter vector, usually the score function. The empirical estimating function is the evaluated estimating function at the data with n observations and the estimated parameters of dimension q. The empirical estimating function is saved in an object called `process` and is used to compute the empirical fluctuation process $W_j(t)$. The test statistics are computed for the partitioning variables by reordering `process` for each z1,...,zl. The advantage is that `process` only have to be computed once in a node. In addition, the p-values are computed. To determine whether there is some overall instability, it is checked whether at least one of the p-values falls below the pre-specified significance level `alpha`. To adjust for multiple testing, the p-values are Bonferroni adjusted, if `bonferroni = TRUE`.

If there is significant instability, the variable z associated with the minimal p-value is used for splitting the node.

Step 3: Split into Nodes

In the third step the observations in the current node should be split for the chosen variable z into B children nodes. In the package party only binary splitting is possible, this means that B = 2. To find the optimal split point a reweight() function is needed to re-fit the model on the same observations but using different weights.

For each possible split point the following steps are conducted in mob(), where obj denotes a fitted model:

```
fmleft <- reweight(obj, weights = weightsleft)
fmright <- reweight(obj, weights = weightsright)
objfun(fmleft) + objfun(fmright)
```

At first for the subsample left from the split point the model is reweight()ed, where in weightsleft the observations in this subsample keep their current weights and those, which are right from the cut point, have zero weights. This means that the parameter estimation only is based on the observations on the left hand side of the split point. The same is conducted for the subsample right from the split point. An objfun() extracts the values of the objective function from the fitted model fmleft and fmright. The sum of both is computed. The objfun() function can be specified in mob_control(), by default it is equal to deviance.

These steps are conducted for all candidate cut points and the one with the minimal sum is chosen.

Step 4: Re-fitting the model

The node is split into children nodes with respect to the chosen split point from step 3. In each node the observations, which enter the first child node, keep their current weights and those observations that go into the other child node receive zero weights and the other way round. The model is re-fitted in both children nodes using the reweight() function.

The procedure is repeated from step 2 as long as no (more) significant parameter instability is detected.

The `mob()` function returns an object of class `mob` inheriting from the class `BinaryTree`. The returned object is a fitted MOB tree, where every node in the tree is connected with a fitted model. Different standard methods can be applied to the fitted MOB tree, if they are available for the fitted `model` class, including `print()`, `predict()`, `residuals()`, `logLik()`, `deviance()`, `weights()`, `coef()` and `summary()`. The `print()`ed MOB tree shows the split points, their test statistics of the parameter instability test and calls the `print()` method for the fitted `model` class in each terminal node. Furthermore, a visualization of the fitted MOB tree via the `plot()` method is possible and in general much easier to interpret. The functions `predict()` and `residuals()` extract the predicted values and the residuals for the terminal nodes, respectively. `logLik()` and `deviance()` compute by default the sum of the log-likelihoods and the sum of the deviances for the fitted models in the terminal nodes, respectively. A `node` argument can be passed to extract the results for any node ID. Note that for the model class `survReg` the `deviance()` function is not available. The functions `weights()`, `coef()` and `summary()` print the results for all terminal nodes. By specifying the `node` argument the results for any node ID can be extracted from the tree. For example, `summary(testmob, node = 4)` returns the summary for the fitted model in node 4. In addition, a function `sctest()` (structural change **test**) is available to extract the results of the parameter instability test. By default the results are printed for all nodes. By passing the `node` argument the results can be returned separately for any node.

3.2. Fitting a MOB Weibull Model with Adjustment for Measurement Error

As already mentioned, a model-based parameter estimation of the Weibull model is integrated in the `mob()` function. To fit a MOB tree based on a Weibull model with adjustment for measurement error a new object of class `StatModel` has to be generated. Especially, the `fit()` function has to be adapted for the new object to conduct a parameter estimation via the corrected log-likelihood, as well as the `reweight()` function. In addition, the `estfun()` has to be modified to integrate the values of the corrected score functions in the parameter instability test. The `objfun()` function has to be adapted as well, because the default setting `objfun = deviance` cannot be applied for the Weibull model. Furthermore, standard methods have to be adapted for the new object, e. g. `print()` and `logLik()`. For the implementation it is important to keep in mind that the package `party` is written object-oriented (S4).

In the following the whole procedure is supported by a data example. The Lung Cancer Data, which is available in the `R` package `survival` including the censored survival data for patients with advanced lung cancer (already mentioned in Section 2.2.1), is used. The relevant variables are:

- `time`: survival time (in days)

- `status`: censoring status (censored $= 1$, dead $= 2$)

- `age`: age in years

- `sex`: (male $= 1$, female $= 2$)

- `ph.ecog`: ECOG performance score (good $= 0$ – dead $= 5$)

- `ph.karno`: Karnofsky performance score (bad $= 0$ – good $= 100$)

- `meal.cal`: calories consumed at meals (assumed to be measured with error)

- `wt.loss`: loss of weight in last six months

New Object `SurvRegcorr` **of class** `StatModel`

For `model = survReg` a Weibull model is considered in the MOB algorithm. `survReg` is of class `StatModel` and consists of five slots: `name` (description for the object), `dpp` (function for data pre-processing), `fit` (a function, which fits the model to the data via `survReg()`), `predict` (a function returning the predicted values for the fitted model; here, `predict` is an empty `function()`) and `capabilities` (consists of two slots, `weights` and `subset` of type logical).

According to `survReg` a new object `SurvRegcorr` of class `StatModel` is implemented to conduct a corrected parameter estimation in the Weibull model:

```
SurvRegcorr <- new("StatModel", name = "Survival Regression with
                corrected log-Likelihood", dpp = ModelEnvFormula,
                capabilities = new("StatModelCapabilities"))
```

The `fit` function is implemented separately and is attached to the new object `SurvRegcorr` via the `@`-operator (`SurvRegcorr@fit`). The new `fit` function provides a corrected model fit for the Weibull model. The whole numbered code for the implemented `fit` function is located in Appendix A.1. In the following the details are described.

A `function` with the following arguments is allocated to `SurvRegcorr@fit` (line 1–2):

object   An object of class `ModelEnvFormula` from package `modeltools`. In `mob()` the object is generated by a function `mobpp()` including the preparation of the model `formula` and the `data` by the function `dpp()`.

weights   An optional vector of weights to be used in the fitting process. By default set to `NULL`.

error.var   A vector of type character. Specifies the variable(s), which is/are subject to measurement error. Only variables included in the `mob()` function as corvariables (in the model `formula` before |) can be considered. Due to practical considerations only continuous variables are considered as `error.var`iables. The partitioning variables are assumed to be error free.

sd.U   A numeric vector including the standard deviation for the error variable(s). Must be of the same lengths as `error.var`.

...   Additional arguments to be passed.

At first, a few error enquiries are conducted (line 5–23). It is checked, if `error.var` and `sd.U` are specified as well as if the type of the `error.var` is `character`, and if `length(sd.U)` is equal to `length(error.var)`. In addition, it is verified, if the `error.var` is one of the passed covariables. If one of these conditions is not fulfilled, the algorithm stops. In line 27–63 the extracted data from `object` is prepared. A new data frame `mydata` is generated, where the variables are re-ordered. The first two columns are the censored survival data, the time variable and status variable. In the next columns follow the variables defined in `error.var`. If there are further error free covariables, they are attached to the data frame behind the error variables. This ordering is conducted, so that the correction for measurement error can be allocated only to the error variables. If `weights` is not equal to `NULL`, only those observations in `mydata` are selected with `weights > 0`. In the case the model is re-fitted with different weights, the parameter estimation is only based on those observations in the current node. In addition, a vector `time` and `event` containing the failure times and the status variable, respectively, as well as the design matrix `A` (see Equation (2.16)) are computed. These values are needed in the log-likelihood of the Weibull model. In line 67–80 the negative corrected log-likelihood of the Weibull model `minus.log.lik.weibull()` is implemented as in Equation (2.58). The value of the corrected negative log-likelihood is returned. In line 84–122 the corrected score functions for β (`score.corr.beta()`) and τ (`score.corr.log.scale()`) from Equation (2.59) and (2.60) are implemented. The model scores of every observation are computed. A $(n \times (q - 1))$-matrix is returned by `score.corr.beta()` and a $(n \times 1)$-matrix by `score.corr.log.scale()`. Both matrixes together are the matrix of the model scores used for the parameter instability test and the robust variance estimator. For computing the corrected log-likelihood and the corrected score functions the moment generating function is needed as well as the derivative of the logarithm of the moment generating function. `M.U()` and `d.log.M.U()` (see line 126–149) are set to 0 for an error free variable and to `(sd.U^2 * betaX^2)/2` and `(sd.U^2 * betaX)` for an `error.var`, respectively. This corresponds to the additive error model with U_i being identically normally distributed with mean zero and variance `sd.U^2`. Multiplying `M.U()` by `1/exp(tau)^2` leads to Equation (2.54), multiplying `d.log.M.U()` by `1/exp(tau)^2` results in Equation (2.55) and multiplying `M.U()` by `-2 * 1/exp(tau)^2` leads to in Equation (2.56).

To compute the corrected parameter estimators, the corrected negative log-likelihood is minimized via the `optim()` function. In the MOB algorithm the objective function should be minimized (see Section 2.2.2, step 2), thus the negative log-likelihood is considered, which is equivalent to maximizing the log-likelihood. For the start values the naive estimators fitted via the `survreg()` function are used (line 153–166). The naive parameter estimates are extracted from the fitted object `survreg.naive`, so that `betaX.start` is equal to `survreg.naive$coef` and `tau.start` is set to `log(survreg.naive$scale)`. The start values are saved in `model.par.naive` and are passed together with `minus.log.lik.weibull` to the `optim()` function (line 170–171):

```
rval <- optim(model.par.naive, minus.log.lik.weibull,
              method = "Nelder-Mead", hessian = TRUE)
```

For optimization the `Nelder-Mead` method is used and the `hessian` matrix is generated. The results of `optim()` are saved in `rval` containing the vector of the corrected parameter estimators for `beta` and `log(scale)`, the `value` of the corrected log-likelihood, the number of iterations (`counts`) and the `hessian` matrix, which is the matrix of the second partial derivatives of the negative corrected log-likelihood. The latter is used for computing the variance of the parameter estimators.

The aim is to wrap the results in a list, so that the returned object of the SurvRegcorr@fit() and the survreg() function are of similar structure and the output of the summary() function of these objects are comparable. Note that only the order of the covariables in the output could be different. In the case of a fitted object via the SurvRegcorr@fit() the columns of the data are re-ordered according to the error variables. The summary of a fitted object via the survreg() function is as follows:

```
Call:
survreg(formula = y ~ ., data = mydata, weights = weights)
                Value Std. Error      z        p
(Intercept)  5.56e+00    0.293256 18.952 4.24e-80
meal.cal     4.28e-05    0.000326  0.131 8.96e-01
Log(scale)  -1.37e-01    0.133833 -1.022 3.07e-01

Scale= 0.872

Weibull distribution
Loglik(model)= -235.8   Loglik(intercept only)= -235.8
        Chisq= 0.02 on 1 degrees of freedom, p= 0.89
Number of Newton-Raphson Iterations: 5
n= 41
```

Thus for the summary of a SurvRegcorr object the parameter estimation and their standard errors to compute the Wald test (z) with p-values are needed. Note that for the scale parameter the inference is done on the log scale to extend the range of the scale parameter from greater than zero to $(-\infty, +\infty)$. Furthermore, the values of the log-likelihood of the full and null model (intercept only) are needed to compute the value of the likelihood ratio test (Chisq) with corresponding p-value. In addition, the number of iterations are printed as well as the sample size n.

In line 176–204 the results are prepared for the returned list. At first, the values of the corrected parameter estimation are extracted from rval and are saved in coef.model. The coefficients coef0 of the null model are extracted from survreg.null, which was fitted in line 157–158 via the survreg() function including only the intercept. A correction for measurement error is not necessary,

because no covariables are included in the model. In line 182–189 the robust
sandwich estimator for covariance matrix of the corrected parameter estimators are
computed. At first, the hessian matrix from `rval` is saved in `hess` (see Equation
(2.63)) and the inverse is computed (`solve(hess)`). In fact, the negative hessian
matrix has to be considered, i. e. the observed Fisher information matrix. Because
of minimizing the negative log-likelihood the sign of the hessian matrix is turned
around. Thus, the negative sign of the hessian matrix is reserved by the negative
sign of the log-likelihood. The value of the corrected `score` function evaluated at
the corrected parameter estimator and their cross product `C` are computed (see
Equation (2.64)). These are used to compute the sandwich estimator `hessinv`
`%*% C %*% hessinv` for the covariance matrix from Equation (2.62). For the scale
parameter the standard error is already considered on the log scale.

In addition, the `linear.predictors`, the `call` function for optimization, the model
`terms` and `ytrans` are computed. In the end a list `z` is generated (line 207–218) and
is returned by the corrected `fit` function. The list includes the following elements:

`coefficients`	the corrected parameter estimators for `beta`
`icoef`	the coefficients of the null model including `intercept` and `log(scale)`
`var`	the robust estimated covariance matrix for the corrected `coefficients` and `log(scale)`
`loglik`	a vector with the value of the log-likelihood of the null model and the value of the corrected log-likelihood. The latter is extracted from the results of the `optim()` function, which returns the value of the negative corrected log-likelihood, thus the value has to be multiplied by minus one.
`iter`	the number of iterations to optimize the corrected log-likelihood
`linear.predictors`	the predicted log survival times ($\hat{\beta}'X$)
`df`	the degrees of freedom (df) of the fitted model
`scale`	the estimated scale parameter. In `rval` the logarithm of the scale parameter is estimated, thus the `exp()` of the estimated `log(scale)` is considered to obtain the `scale` parameter.

idf   the degrees of freedom of the null model. They are needed for the likelihood ratio test as well as the degrees of freedom df of the fitted model. The difference of both are the degrees of freedom for the likelihood ratio test.

df.residuals   the degrees of freedom of the residuals. They are computed by the difference between the sample size n and df

terms   the model terms are taken from survreg.naive

means   the mean of the covariables

call   the function call for optimization

dist   the underlying distribution of the model fit, here the weibull distribution

ytrans   the transformed response variable ytrans including the log survival time and the status variable

error.var   the vector of error variables passed to the model

sd.U   the standard deviation(s) of the error variable(s). error.var and sd.U are needed for the reweight() function.

emp.estfun.corr   a $(n \times q)$-matrix containing the values of score.corr.beta() and score.corr.log.scale() evaluated at the observed data and the corrected parameter estimators extracted from rval$par. This model scores are needed for the fluctuation test (of which more later).

According to the fit function of an object of class survReg in line 220–224 the object is saved in ModelEnv and the weights vector is saved in weights. If additional arguments are passed, they are saved in addargs. In the end the generated list z is allocated to two classes, SurvRegcorr and survreg. This is important, so that further (generic) functions can be implemented for the new object and functions, which are already available for an object of class survreg, can be inherited to an object of class SurvRegcorr, such as the summary() function.

The new object SurvRegcorr of class StatModel can be used to fit a MOB Weibull model with correction for measurement error. For the Lung Cancer Data the function call is as follows:

```
testmob <- mob(Surv(time,status) ~ meal.cal | ph.ecog + ph.karno +
               age + sex + wt.loss, data = lung, control = ctrl,
               model = SurvRegcorr, error.var = c("meal.cal"),
               sd.U = 0.2)
```

with

```
ctrl <- mob_control(alpha = 0.05, bonferroni = TRUE, minsplit = 40,
            objfun = function(object) {-as.vector(logLik(object))},
            verbose = TRUE)
```

In the model `formula` the response variable, consisting of `time` and `status`, is specified via the `Surv()` function. `meal.cal` as the only covariable and a total of five partitioning variables are passed to `mob()`. A model of class `SurvRegcorr` is fitted, thus the `error.variable` `meal.cal` with `sd.U = 0.2` (an arbitrary choice) is specified for the `SurvRegcorr@fit()` function. In `crtl` the control parameters are saved. The significance level `alpha` and `bonferroni` are set to the default values. The minimal sample size `minsplit` is set to 40 and `verbose` to `TRUE`. `objfun` is modified to the negative log-likelihood. The result of this function call for the Lung Cancer data is a fitted MOB tree and is shown in Figure 3.1. The new implemented `fit()` function (`SurvRegcorr@fit()`) is used to fit the specified model `SurvRegcorr` (Weibull model with adjustment for measurement error) with `formula = Surv(time,status)` $\sim$ `meal.cal | ph.ecog + ph.karno + age + sex + wt.loss` for all observations in the current node, respectively. The survival time (in days) is split with respect to `ph.ecog` (good $= 0$ – dead $= 5$) less or equal to 1 and greater than 1.

A modified `print()` function is implemented to generate an output for an object of class `SurvRegcorr` including the value of the corrected estimated coefficients and scale parameter. According to `print.survReg()` from package `modeltools`, the `print()` function, where `x` is a fitted Weibull model of class `SurvRegcorr`, is as follows:

```
print.SurvRegcorr <- function (x, digits = max(3,
                               getOption("digits") - 3), ...) {
    dist <- x$dist
    substr(dist, 1, 1) <- toupper(substr(dist, 1, 1))
    cat(paste("Corrected", dist, "survival regression",
    paste("(scale = ", paste(format(x$scale, digits = digits),
    sep = ", "),")", sep = ""), "with coefficients:\n"))
    print.default(format(coef(x), digits = digits), print.gap = 2,
        quote = FALSE)
    invisible(x)
}
```

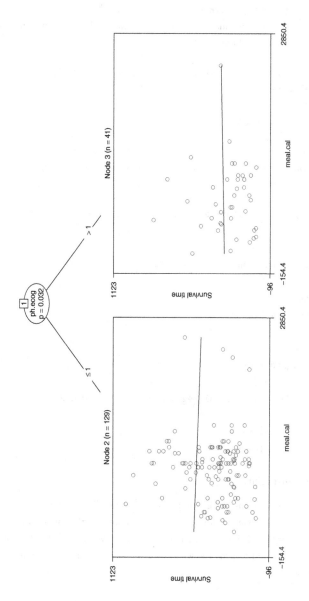

Figure 3.1.: Model-based recursive partitioning with Lung Cancer Data

In comparison to print.survReg() only a "Corrected" is added to make clear that a corrected parameter estimation is conducted. In the data example an output of the following structure is printed:

```
Corrected Weibull survival regression (scale = 0.8722)
with coefficients:
Intercept    meal.cal
5.558e+00   4.281e-05
```

The print()ed fitted MOB tree testmob shows the split points, their test statistics of the parameter instability test and calls the print.SurvRegcorr() function in each terminal node:

```
1) ph.ecog <= 1; criterion = 0.968, statistic = 18.172
  2)*  weights = 129
Terminal node model
Corrected Weibull survival regression (scale = 0.68)
with coefficients:
 Intercept     meal.cal
 6.204e+00   -4.573e-05


1) ph.ecog > 1
  3)*  weights = 41
Terminal node model
Corrected Weibull survival regression (scale = 0.8722)
with coefficients:
Intercept    meal.cal
5.558e+00   4.281e-05
```

Parameter Instability

To compute the parameter instability test the mob() function requires an extractor function estfun() and weights(). The weights() function for the new object SurvRegcorr is implemented according to weights.survReg() from package modeltools and returns the weights of the observations in a fitted object of class SurvRegcorr:

```
weights.SurvRegcorr <- function (object, ...)
{
    if (is.null(object$weights))
        rep(1, NROW(residuals(object)))
    else object$weights
}
```

`estfun.SurvRegcorr()` returns the empirical estimating function from the fitted model, where `x` is a fitted model of class `SurvRegcorr`:

```
estfun.SurvRegcorr <- function (x, ...)
{
    rval <- x$emp.estfun.corr
    return(rval)
}
```

The returned value `emp.estfun.corr` is a $(n \times q)$-matrix containing the values of the corrected score functions for β and τ as defined in Equation (2.59) and (2.60) evaluated at the observed data and the corrected parameter estimators. `emp.estfun.corr` is already computed in the `SurvRegcorr@fit()` function. From `x` only the values of the empirical estimating function have to be extracted via the $-operator. Actually, the negative score functions are considered. However, the negative sign does not influence the result of the parameter instability test and therefore it can be omitted.

Two approaches for implementation of the `estfun()` were considered: Compute `emp.estfun.corr` in `SurvRegcorr@fit` or in `estfun()`. Both approaches lead to the same results. It was decided for the first version, because the needed values such as the design matrix `A`, the `time` and `event` vector as well as the moment generating function `M.U()` are already generated in `SurvRegcorr@fit` and can be easily used for computing the empirical estimating function.

The empirical estimating function is saved in an object called `process` and is used to compute the empirical fluctuation process $W_j(t)$ (see Equation (2.75)), where `process` corresponds to $\hat{\psi}_{corr}$. Thus, the correction for measurement error is integrated in the test statistic via the modified `estfun.SurvRegcorr()`. The advantage is that `emp.estfun.corr` only has to be computed once in a node.

For the data example, the R output of the parameter instability test for `verbose = TRUE` in `mob_control()` is shown in the following:

```
------------------------------------------
Fluctuation tests of splitting variables:
             ph.ecog    ph.karno          age         sex    wt.loss
statistic 18.17169330 16.4570006 12.2002663 12.4410963 4.6393177
p.value    0.03157357  0.0635349  0.3115919  0.2877806 0.9990544

Best splitting variable: ph.ecog
Perform split? yes
------------------------------------------


Node properties:
ph.ecog <= 1; criterion = 0.968, statistic = 18.172


------------------------------------------
Fluctuation tests of splitting variables:
            ph.ecog   ph.karno          age       sex    wt.loss
statistic 2.4530458 3.2982287 7.0827317 2.7462348 7.0650369
p.value   0.9999996 0.9999277 0.8678298 0.9999965 0.8696493

Best splitting variable: age
Perform split? no
------------------------------------------
```

The p-values are Bonferroni adjusted at a level of alpha = 0.05, because in mob_control() bonferroni is set to TRUE. The test statistic and the p-value is printed for each partitioning variable. The first time of conducting the test of parameter instability the variable ph.ecog has the smallest p-value and is chosen for splitting. The second time no more parameter instability is detected, i. e. the p-value of age does not fall below the significance level alpha, and the algorithm stops. In addition, the split point for ph.ecog is shown (ph.ecog <= 1), of which more in the next passage. This output reflects the results of the plot in Figure 3.1.

Optimal Split Point

To find the optimal split point the negative log-likelihood is considered, i. e. objfun = function(object) -as.vector(logLik(object)), which is specified in mob_control(). To extract the value of the corrected log-likelihood, the

logLik() function has to be defined for the new object SurvRegcorr. According to
logLik.survReg() from package modeltools the function logLik.SurvRegcorr(),
where object is a fitted model of class SurvRegcorr, is given as follows:

```
logLik.SurvRegcorr <- function (object, ...)
{
    structure(object$loglik[2], df = NCOL(object$var),
                                    class = "logLik")
}
```

logLik.SurvRegcorr() extracts the value of the corrected log-likelihood and the
number of estimated parameters in the model (df = degrees of freedom). The generic
function AIC can be applied to a SurvRegcorr object as well ($\rightarrow$AIC.logLik()).
In the data example the function calls and the returned values are as follows:

```
> logLik(testmob)
'log Lik.' -853.8164 (df=7)

> AIC(testmob)
[1] 1721.633
```

In addition, the reweight() function has to be adapted for the new object
SurvRegcorr, thus the fitted model is reweight()ed via the corrected fit function
SurvRegcorr@fit(), where object is a fitted model object of class SurvRegcorr
and weights is a vector of weights:

```
reweight.SurvRegcorr <- function (object, weights, ... )
{
    fit <- SurvRegcorr@fit
    do.call("fit", c(list(object = object$ModelEnv,
    weights = weights, error.var = object$error.var,
    sd.U = object$sd.U), object$addargs))
}
```

This function is implemented according to reweight.survReg() from package
party. The modification is that fit is set to SurvRegcorr@fit, thus a re-fitted
model object is returned with corrected parameter estimators. To find the optimal
cut point the fitted model is reweight()ed for each candidate split point. For a
possible split point the following is computed:

```
fmleft <- reweight(obj, weights = weightsleft)
fmright <- reweight(obj, weights = weightsright)
-logLik(fmleft) + -logLik(fmright)
```

The last line correspond to the partitioned corrected log-likelihood in Equation (2.78), where $\sum_{i \in L(\xi)} \Psi_{corr}\left(Y_i, \hat{\vartheta}^{(L)*}\right)$ conform to -logLik(fmleft) and $\sum_{i \in R(\xi)} \Psi_{corr}\left(Y_i, \hat{\vartheta}^{(R)*}\right)$ to -logLik(fmright).

In the following an overview of the MOB algorithm (see Section 2.2.2) in R for the Weibull model with adjustment for measurement error is given:

1. The SurvRegcorr model with given formula is fitted with all observations of the current node via the SurvRegcorr@fit() function.

2. A test for parameter instability is conducted, where the values of the corrected score functions are extracted via estfun.SurvRegcorr() to compute the test statistics for each partitioning variable. weights.SurvRegcorr() extracts the weights to determine which observations are in the current node. If there is some overall instability, select the variable z associated with the minimal p-value falls below the significance level alpha. Adjusted p-values are returned for bonferroni = TRUE.

3. Compute the optimal split point for the partitioning variable z, which minimizes objfun(fmleft) + objfun(fmright). objfun is set to -logLik(), where logLik.SurvRegcorr() extracts the value of the corrected log-likelihood from the reweight()ed model for every possible candidate split point.

4. Split the nodes into children nodes with respect to the cut point from step 3 and re-fit the models in the children nodes via the reweight.SurvRegcorr() function.

mob() is conducted as long as in step 2 no further p-value falls below the significance level alpha, i. e. no more parameter instability can be detected.

For the fitted MOB tree several standard methods are inherited if they are available for the fitted model. Thus, for the new object SurvRegcorr further generic functions have to be adapted.

SurvRegcorr is an object of class SurvRegcorr and survreg. As already described

above `print.SurvRegcorr()`, `logLik.SurvRegcorr()` (thus `AIC.logLik()`, too)
and `weights.SurvRegcorr()` are implemented for the object `SurvRegcorr`. In addition, `SurvRegcorr` inherits the functions `predict()`, `residuals()`, `coef()` by
`survreg` as well as the generic function `summary()` (i. e. `summary.SurvRegcorr()`
$\rightarrow$ `summary.survreg()`), thus the summary structure is the same as for a `survreg`
object.

Hence, all the standard methods described in the section before can be applied for
the fitted MOB tree via `mob()` with `model = SurvRegcorr` as well as the `plot()`
function to visualise the tree.

For the Lung Cancer data the summary for the `testmob` in the terminal node with
node ID 3 (`summary(testmob, node=3)`) is given by

```
Call:
optim(model.par.naive, minus.log.lik.weibull,
      method = "Nelder-Mead", hessian = TRUE)
                Value Std. Error      z         p
Intercept     5.56e+00  0.222138 25.020 3.72e-138
meal.cal      4.28e-05  0.000148  0.289  7.73e-01
Log(scale)   -1.37e-01  0.208757 -0.655  5.12e-01

Scale= 0.872

Weibull distribution
Loglik(model)= -235.8   Loglik(intercept only)= -235.8
        Chisq= 0.02 on 1 degrees of freedom, p= 0.89
Number of Newton-Raphson Iterations: 90
n= 41
```

The structure is equal to the summary of an object of class `survreg`. Different is
the `Call`, because the corrected log-likelihood is fitted via the `optim()` function
and not via the `survreg()` function. In comparison to the output of the `print`
method, further information is given, such as the estimated robust standard errors
for the corrected parameter estimators, the test statistics of the Wald test and the
corresponding p-values. The value of the corrected log-likelihood and the value of
the likelihood of the null model are printed. From that the value of the likelihood
ratio test (`Chisq`) with p-value is computed.

Three problems arise by fitting a MOB Weibull model via the `mob()` function
with `model = SurvRegcorr`:

1. In comparison to the fit function `survreg()` the `optim()` function has a
   longer running time. By optimizing the corrected log-likelihood via the
   `optim()` function the running time is extended for fitting the MOB.

2. If the start values for the `optim()` function are varied, different parameter
   estimators result. By setting the start values to the naive estimators, the
   `optim()` algorithm should be already close to the true optimum and the risk
   should be reduced to end up in a local extremum.

3. In the third step the fitted model is `reweight()`ed for every possible split
   point to find the optimal split point. This means for example for a metric
   partitioning variable **age** of the Lung Cancer Data:
   First age is `sort()`ed and the double values are eliminated via the `unique()`
   function (`sort(unique(lung$age))`). Assuming **age** has 40 different values.
   For every value (= possible split point) the data is split with respect to the split
   point and is `reweight()`ed for both subsamples. The sum of the partitioned
   corrected log-likelihood is saved in `dev[i]`, so that for 40 different values of
   age the `reweight()` function is conducted 80 times. At the same time, this
   means that the `optim()` function is called every time, when `reweight()` is
   conducted, therefore the running time is extended seriously.
   In the case of a categorical partitioning variable the problem is less serious,
   because the possible split points are only a few and in the case of a binary
   splitting variable the split point is already clear. Thus, the running time
   of `mob()` depends on the model complexity as well as how many nodes are
   detected and which types of partitioning variables are selected for splitting.

4. Simulation Study

The aim of the simulation study is to analyse the performance of the corrected estimator, which is derived via the new implemented corrected log-likelihood of the Weibull model. The simulation study is divided in three parts. At first, the behaviour of the new implemented `fit` function `SurvRegcorr@fit()`, which is used in the MOB algorithm, is analysed separately (see Section 4.1). Secondly, the performance of `SurvRegcorr@fit()` within the MOB algorithm as well as the detection rate for the true underlying tree structure is examined (see Section 4.2). Thirdly, the prediction accuracy of a global model and a MOB are compared (see Section 4.3). In all parts the following four approaches are considered:

1. Benchmark estimation

2. Naive estimation

3. Regression calibration

4. Corrected estimation via the corrected log-likelihood.

The benchmark estimator is the maximum of the log-likelihood (see Equation 2.48) including the usually unobservable true covariable V_i. The naive estimator is obtained by substituting the error-prone covariable W_i for V_i in the log-likelihood from Equation (2.48), which means that the measurement error is ignored. In the case of the regression calibration W_i is substituted by the estimate $\hat{\tilde{\mu}}_i$ (see Equation (2.10)) of the conditional expectation $\mathbb{E}(V_i|W_i)$. For these three approaches the `survreg()` function from the package `survial` with `dist = "weibull"` is used to optimize the log-likelihood. The corrected estimation is the maximum of the corrected log-likelihood derived in Equation (2.58). In R the corrected estimator is computed via the new implemented `SurvRegcorr@fit()` function.

Thereby, the simulation parameters

- `size` (sample size),

- **sd.U** (standard deviation of the measurement error),

- **beta.true** (true value(s) of the parameter estimator(s)),

- **tau.true** (log-transformed shape parameter of the Weibull distribution and log scale parameter of the Weibull model),

- and **prop.cens** (amount of censorship)

are varied. For all three parts of the simulation study the sample **size** is set to 100, 500 and 1000. The standard deviation of the measurement error **sd.U** is set to 0, 0.1, 0.4 and 0.8. If **sd.U** = 0, the estimation of β_V for the naive approach, regression calibration and corrected approach are equal to the benchmark estimation, because no measurement errors influence the estimation. The amount of censorship **prop.cens** is set to 0% (no censoring) as well as to approximately 35% and 65%. The values of **beta.true** and **tau.true** do depend on the part of the simulation study. By choosing different values for **beta.true** and **tau.true** the distribution of the failure time is varied. The distribution of the true covariable V_i is assumed to be normal. In the first part of the simulation study the performance of the four different approaches are also analysed for V_i uniformly distributed. The estimation is repeated 1000 times in the first part, 500 times in the second and in the third part. For every cell of the simulation grid the results are presented in tables plus they are visualized in boxplots, where **beta.true** and **tau.true** are drawn in the boxplots as a horizontal line. For some constellations of the simulation parameters and simulated data, the **optim()** function used in the **SurvRegcorr@fit()** function does not converge or the resulting hessian matrix is singular, so that the inverse of this matrix cannot be computed. Therefore, the **SurvRegcorr@fit()** function is modified for the simulation study, in that way that error warnings are absorbed not to interrupt the simulation runs. The modified **SurvRegcorr@fit()** function is saved in **SurvRegcorr.sim.r**. In the following only selected results are presented.

4.1. Check the **fit** Function

At first, the new implemented **fit** function **SurvRegcorr@fit()** is analysed separately to check how this function adjusts for biased parameter estimation in the case of covariates with measurement error. The resulting corrected estimators are compared to the benchmark and naive estimators as well as to the corrected estimators obtained by the regression calibration.

4.1.1. Check the `fit` Function - only W

Under the assumption of an additive measurement error model $W_i = V_i + U_i$ with $U_i \sim N(0, \sigma_U^2)$ (i. e. homoscedastic normal errors) and $U_i \perp \{T_i, V_i, C_i\}$ (see Section 2.1.1), a data set is simulated, which is used to estimate the model parameters in the different approaches and to compare the performance between each other. For the beginning, only one covariate, which is subject to measurement error, is considered. Thus, the data set consists of the failure times and the censoring indicator as well as the error-prone covariate. In R random numbers are generated:

1. The covariable for a fixed value of σ_U^2:

   - True covariable: $V_i \sim N(0, 1)$ (`V <-rnorm(size,0,1)`)
     or $V_i \sim Unif(0, \sqrt{12})$ with $sd(V_i) = 1$ (`V <-runif(size,0,sqrt(12))`)
   - Measurement error: $U_i \sim N(0, \sigma_U^2)$ (`U <-rnorm(size,0,sd.U)`)
   - $\rightarrow W_i = V_i + U_i$

2. The values of the response variable are the censored failure times, denoted by $\tilde{Y}_i = (min(T_i, C_i), \delta_i)$. A random censorship is assumed ($C_i \perp \{T_i, V_i\}$), where the proportion of censoring is varied. For a given β_V (`beta.true`), τ (`tau.true`) and each covariable value V_i, a failure time is generated from the Weibull distribution. The failure time T_i is derived via the distribution function $F(T_i)$. If T_i is a random number, then $D_i = F(T_i)$ is uniformly distributed in $[0, 1]$. If $D_i \sim Unif(0, 1)$, then $(1 - D_i) \sim Unif(0, 1)$ holds, too (cf. Bender et al., 2005). To generate the censored failure times $\tilde{Y}_i$ the following steps are conducted:

   - Failure time: Using the relationships from above, T_i is derived as

   $$T_i = [-log(D_i) \cdot exp(\beta_V' V_i / exp(\tau))]^{exp(\tau)} \text{ with } D_i \sim Unif(0, 1).$$

   The derivation is located in Appendix B.7.

   - Censoring time: Since C_i is independent of $\beta_V' V_i$, the censoring variable is generated from an uniform distribution. `C <- runif(size, min = 0, max = b.cens)`, where `b.cens` is chosen in such a way that the proportion of censoring is controlled.

   - $\rightarrow \delta_i = 0$, if $T_i > C_i$ (censored) and $\delta_i = 1$, if $T_i \leq C_i$ (event)

   - $\rightarrow \tilde{Y}_i = (min(T_i, C_i), \delta_i)$

The simulated data set is used to estimate the model parameters. The different
approaches are computed in R in the following way:

- Benchmark estimation:
  `survreg(Surv(time,status)` $\sim$ `V, data = data, dist = "weibull")`

- Naive estimation:
  `survreg(Surv(time,status)` $\sim$ `W, data = data, dist = "weibull")`

- Regression calibration:
  `survreg(Surv(time,status)` $\sim$ `W.reg.calib, data = data,`
  `dist = "weibull"),`
  where `W.reg.calib` are the conditional expectations, computed as in Equation
  (2.10).

- Corrected estimation:
  `SurvRegcorr@fit(object, weights = NULL, error.var = error.var,`
  `sd.U = sd.U)`
  with `object = Surv(time,status)`$\sim$ `W, error.var = c("W")` and `sd.U` is
  set to the value of the present cell of the simulation grid.

The simulation grid and especially the values for `beta.true` and `tau.true` are
given in Table 4.1. Negative and positive values for `beta.true` are considered
in combination with an increasing and decreasing hazard rate. If τ is smaller
than zero, $\nu = exp(\tau)$ is smaller than one. Thus, for `tau.true` = -0.3 the hazard
rate given by $h(t) = \frac{1}{\nu} \cdot t^{1/\nu-1}$ (see Equation (2.37)) is increasing. If τ is greater
than zero, $\nu = exp(\tau)$ is greater than one. This means that for `tau.true` = 0.5 a
decreasing hazard rate is simulated. The whole procedure is repeated 1000 times,
specified in `monte.carlo` (abbreviated `mc`). For the repeated estimation the sample
mean of the parameter estimators

$$\bar{\hat{\beta}} = \frac{1}{mc} \sum_{j=1}^{mc} \hat{\beta}_j, \qquad (4.1)$$

the sample standard deviation

$$sd(\hat{\beta}) = \sqrt{\frac{1}{mc} \sum_{j=1}^{mc} \left(\hat{\beta}_j - \bar{\hat{\beta}} \right)}, \qquad (4.2)$$

size	sd.U	beta.true	tau.true	prop.cens
100	0	-0.2	-0.3	0%
500	0.1			35%
1000	0.4			65%
	0.8	-0.2	0.5	0%
				35%
				65%
		0.4	-0.3	0%
				35%
				65%
		0.4	0.5	0%
				35%
				65%

Table 4.1.: Simulation grid for *Check the fit Function* with $\tilde{Y} \sim W$ and monte.carlo = 1000

the average of the standard deviation estimators

$$\overline{sd(\hat{\beta})} = \frac{1}{mc} \sum_{j=1}^{mc} sd_j^*, \tag{4.3}$$

with $sd^* = \sqrt{I^{-1}(\cdot)C(\cdot)I^{-1}(\cdot)}$ (see Equation (2.62)) in the case of the corrected approach and otherwise $sd^* = \sqrt{I^{-1}(\cdot)}$, are calculated. The calculation of the sample and mean standard deviation is conducted to check the estimation of the implemented sandwich estimator for the corrected approach. These two quantities should result in comparable estimators. The mean squared error (MSE) is obtained as follows

$$\widehat{MSE} = \frac{1}{mc} \sum_{j=1}^{mc} (\hat{\beta}_j - \beta_{true})^2. \tag{4.4}$$

An approximate confidence interval

$$\hat{\beta}_j \pm z_{1-\alpha/2} \cdot sd_j^* \tag{4.5}$$

is computed in each replication, where $z_{1-\alpha/2}$ is the $(1 - \alpha/2)$-quantile of the standard normal distribution. It is counted, how many times the true parameter beta.true lies within the boundaries of the confidence interval, in the following referred to as *coverage probability*. If the approximate normal distribution, which is assumed for the calculation of the confidence interval in Equation (4.5), is fulfilled, the coverage probability should be around 95%.

The same is computed for the log scale parameter of the Weibull model replacing β by τ. In addition, the mean expected failure time is considered

$$\widehat{\mathbb{E}(T|V)} = exp(\hat{\beta}'_V \bar{V})\Gamma(exp(\hat{\tau}) + 1), \tag{4.6}$$

to see how the differences between the resulting parameter estimates affect the expected failure time. The derivation is given in Appendix B.8.

As already mentioned for some constellations of the simulation parameters and simulated data, problems with the optimization occur. In these cases, the parameter estimators cannot be computed and are set to `NA`. A variable `count.NA` is introduced, which counts the number of failed optimizations. The averages and the standard deviation in Equations (4.1) – (4.4) as well as the coverage probability only base on those observations, where the optimization does not fail, i. e. `mc = monte.carlo - count.NA`.

Results

In the following two constellations of the simulation grid of Table 4.1 are presented in detail. Starting with `beta.true = -0.2`, `tau.true = -0.3`, `prob.cens = 35%` and normally distributed V_i: The results for sample size 100, 500 and 1000 are presented in Appendix C.1.1. The boxplots of $\hat{\beta}_V$ and $\hat{\tau}$ for sample size 100 are depicted in Figure C.1 and C.2, respectively. In the case of `sd.U = 0` and `sd.U = 0.1` the resulting boxplots of $\hat{\beta}_V$ are nearly the same and the sample median is equal to `beta.true` for all approaches. Considering `sd.U = 0.4` the sample median of the regression calibration and of the corrected estimators is comparable to the benchmark estimation. However, they show a wider range of variation. The boxplot of the naive estimators is shifted upwards. Since `beta.true` is negative, the absolute value has to be considered. This means that for the naive estimation the effect of β_V is attenuated. In the case of `sd.U = 0.8` the naive estimator, the regression calibration and the corrected estimator show one outlier, thus the presentation of the boxplots is compressed. The boxplots and the sample median of $\hat{\tau}$ are similar for `sd.U = 0`, `sd.U = 0.1` and `sd.U = 0.4`, where `tau.true` is overestimated for all approaches. As for $\hat{\beta}_V$ in the boxplot of `sd.U = 0.8` outliers for the naive estimator, regression calibration and corrected estimator were generated. In Figure C.3 – C.6 the results of sample size 500 and 1000 are shown. The boxplots of $\hat{\beta}_V$ with `sd.U = 0` and `sd.U = 0.1` are similar to those of 100. Again, for sd.U = 0.4 and sd.U = 0.8 the sample median of the benchmark estimator, regression calibration and corrected estimator are almost equal to beta.true. No outliers are generated for sd.U = 0.8. All in all, the attenuation for the naive estimator becomes more apparent.

For sd.U = 0 and sd.U = 0.1 the resulting boxplots of $\hat{\tau}$ are almost equal for all approaches and the sample median of the estimates are equal to tau.true. In the case of sd.U = 0.4 and sd.U = 0.8 the sample median of the naive estimation is equal to the benchmark estimation and quite close to tau.true. In comparison to the benchmark estimation the sample median of the naive and regression calibration are shifted a little upwards. The variation range is comparable for all approaches. The summary tables are located in Table C.1 - C.3 for sample size 100, 500 and 1000. The sample mean $(\bar{\hat{\beta}}_V)$ and median $(med(\hat{\beta}_V))$ of the repeated estimation as well as the sample standard deviation $(sd(\hat{\beta}_V))$ and the mean of the estimated standard deviations $(\overline{sd(\hat{\beta}_V)})$ are shown. Furthermore, the coverage probability $(\% \in \text{CI})$, the mean squared error $(\widehat{MSE})$ and the expected failure time $(\widehat{\mathbb{E}(T)})$ are presented. For the calculation see Equation (4.1) – (4.6). The same quantities are shown for $\hat{\tau}$. In the column of the expected failure times the number of NAs (#NA) is presented that is equal to the number of failed optimizations. Starting with sample size 100 and β_V (see Table C.1): $\bar{\hat{\beta}}_V$ and $med(\hat{\beta}_V)$ are almost the same within each approach and error standard deviation, except sd.U = 0.8, because of the outliers as already seen in the boxplots. $sd(\hat{\beta}_V)$ and $\overline{sd(\hat{\beta}_V)}$ are (almost) equal for sd.U = 0, sd.U = 0.1 and sd.U = 0.4 for every approach, respectively. For the corrected estimation $\overline{sd(\hat{\beta}_V)}$ is smaller than $sd(\hat{\beta}_V)$. Here, the sandwich estimation underestimates the standard deviation, this is overcome by increasing sample size. This suggests that for an increasing sample size the implemented sandwich estimator for the corrected approach moves closer to the true variation. For sd.U = 0.8 $sd(\hat{\beta}_V)$ and $\overline{sd(\hat{\beta}_V)}$ show different values, except the benchmark estimation, here the quantities are equal. For the naive estimation and regression calibration $sd(\hat{\beta}_V)$ is larger than $\overline{sd(\hat{\beta}_V)}$. For the corrected estimation an artefact with $sd(\hat{\beta}) = 755512$ is generated. These differences are traced back to the outliers (cf. Figure C.1). For sd.U = 0 and sd.U = 0.1 the estimated sample standard deviation does not differ for the four approaches. In the case of sd.U = 0.4 the standard deviation for the regression calibration and the corrected estimator is higher compared to the benchmark estimator. The naive estimator shows the lowest standard deviation.

Considering sd.U = 0 and sd.U = 0.1 the coverage probability of the benchmark estimation is equal to 96.6% and 95%, this suggests that here the assumption of the normal distribution is justified. The regression calibration and naive approach show (almost) equal values compared to the benchmark estimation. The coverage probability of the corrected estimators lies a little below the one of the benchmark estimation. Considering sd.U = 0.4 the coverage probability of the regression calibration with 94.4% and of the benchmark estimation with 94.5% are comparable. The corrected estimation has a lower coverage probability with 93.3% than the benchmark approach and the naive estimation shows the lowest value with 91.3%. For sd.U = 0.8 the probability of the corrected estimation is comparable to the benchmark estimation with 95.6%. The regression calibration has a little lower coverage probability than the benchmark estimation. For the naive estimation the probability decreases further to 80.7%. $\widehat{MSE}$ is the same for sd.U = 0 as well as for sd.U = 0.1 and rather small. For sd.U = 0.4 the MSE of the regression calibration and corrected estimation is only a little higher than the MSE of the benchmark estimation. The naive estimation shows the lowest MSE. In the case of sd.U = 0.8 the MSE of the naive estimation, regression calibration and corrected estimation, is increased compared to the benchmark estimation, where the regression calibration shows the highest and naive approach the lowest value. The expected failure time $\widehat{\mathbb{E}(T)}$ results in equal values for sd.U = 0 and sd.U = 0.1, respectively. In the case of sd.U = 0.4 and sd.U = 0.8 the expected failure time of the corrected estimation is equal to the value of the benchmark estimation. For the regression calibration and naive estimation $\widehat{\mathbb{E}(T)}$ differs from the benchmark estimation.

The results for $\hat{\tau}$ do not differ strongly for the different approaches in the case of sd.U = 0, sd.U = 0.1 and sd.U = 0.4. For sd.U = 0.8 the results are skewed due to the outliers (cf. Figure C.2). The optimization only failed in 6 of 1000 cases for the corrected estimation with sd.U = 0.8.

The summary tables of sample size 500 and 1000 are shown in Table C.2 and C.3. All in all, the variance and the MSE of $\hat{\beta}_V$ and $\hat{\tau}$ is decreasing for increasing sample size. The coverage probability of beta.true for sd.U = 0 and sd.U = 0.1 is nearly the same for all approaches, respectively. For sd.U = 0.4 and sd.U = 0.8 the coverage probability of the corrected and regression calibration is comparable to the benchmark estimation. The probability of the naive estimation is decreasing for increasing sample size. $\widehat{\mathbb{E}(T)}$ is equal for all approaches with sd.U = 0, sd.U = 0.1 and sd.U = 0.4. In the case of sd.U = 0.8 the corrected and benchmark estimation have the same values of $\widehat{\mathbb{E}(T)}$. The naive estimation and regression calibration result in a little higher values. For $\hat{\tau}$ the results for all approaches and sd.Us are comparable, no noticeable differences is observed. In total, no optimization fail for sample size 500 and 1000.

The results for $V_i \sim Unif(0, \sqrt{12})$ do not differ from those with $V_i \sim N(0,1)$ as described above (cf. Appendix C.1.2). As V_i is uniformly distributed in $[0, \sqrt{12}]$ the range of V_i differs from a standard normally distributed V_i. Therefore, the values of $\widehat{\mathbb{E}(T)}$ are different from those with $V_i \sim N(0,1)$, because the mean value of V_i is substituted in $\widehat{\mathbb{E}(T)}$.

The estimation accuracy for 0% and 65% censoring are quite similar to the results described above with 35% censoring. Only for 65% censoring more problems with outliers and with the convergence of the optimization in all approaches occur.

The constellation beta.true $= 0.4$ and tau.true $= -0.3$ of the simulation grid perform in the same way with respect to the estimation accuracy of the different approaches (see CD, attached to the appendix). For the corrected estimation problems with the optimization for sd.U $= 0.8$ and sample size 100 occur again. For 65% censoring and sample size 100 outliers are generated.

The results of beta.true $= 0.4$, tau.true $= 0.5$, prob.cens $= 0\%$ and normally distributed V_i are shown in Appendix C.1.3 for sample size 100, 500 and 1000. In Figure C.13 and C.14 the boxplots of $\hat{\beta}_V$ and $\hat{\tau}$ for sample size 100 are depicted. Considering sd.U $= 0$ the results of $\hat{\beta}_V$ for all four approaches are the same, as it should be and the sample median is almost equal to beta.true. For sd.U $= 0.1$ the results are quite similar to the one with no measurement error. In the case of sd.U $= 0.4$ and sd.U $= 0.8$ the benchmark estimator, the regression calibration and the corrected estimator are nearly the same. The corrected estimator shows a little more variation. As expected the naive estimator is shifted downwards, for sd.U $= 0.8$ more than for sd.U $= 0.4$.

The resulting boxplots of $\hat{\tau}$ for sd.U $= 0$, sd.U $= 0.1$ and sd.U $= 0.4$ are similar (see Figure C.14). The true value of τ is underestimated for both error standard deviations. The range of variation is higher for sd.U $= 0.1$ and for sd.U $= 0.4$ compared to sd.U $= 0$. Considering sd.U $= 0.8$, the benchmark estimator and the corrected estimator have nearly the same sample median, but the variation of the corrected estimator is larger. The sample median of the naive and the regression calibration estimator lies a little over the benchmark estimator, but closer to tau.true.

The results of sample size 500 and 1000 are comparable (cf. Figure C.15, C.16,

C.17 and C.18) to those of sample size 100. For sd.U = 0.4 and sd.U = 0.8 the
sample median of $\hat{\tau}$ moves closer to tau.true. Moreover, the attenuation of the
naive estimator of β_V as well as for the naive estimator of τ and the regression
calibration for τ becomes more apparent for increasing sample size.

In Table C.7 – C.9 the summary tables of $\hat{\beta}_V$ and $\hat{\tau}$ are presented in detail for
sample size 100, 500 and 1000. Starting with sample size 100 and β_V (see Table
C.7): $\bar{\hat{\beta}}_V$ and $med(\hat{\beta}_V)$ result in comparable estimation within every approach
and for all sd.Us, which is a sign of no noticeable outliers. $\widehat{sd(\hat{\beta}_V)}$ is smaller than
$sd(\hat{\beta}_V)$. Again, the sandwich estimation underestimates the standard deviation,
this is overcome by increasing sample size. For sd.U = 0 and sd.U = 0.1 the
sample standard deviation is nearly the same for all four approaches, respectively.
For sd.U = 0.4 and sd.U = 0.8 $sd(\hat{\beta}_V)$ of the regression calibration and corrected
estimation is higher in comparison to the benchmark estimation, respectively. The
difference is stronger for sd.U = 0.8 than for sd.U = 0.4. Noticeable is that
$sd(\hat{\beta}_V)$ of the naive estimator is the lowest one. The coverage probability ($\% \in$ CI)
of the benchmark estimation varies around 94 - 95%. The coverage probability of
the corrected estimators turns out to be smaller than for the benchmark estimation.
The coverage probability of the regression calibration is comparable to the benchmark estimation. Only for sd.U = 0.8 it is a little lower. For sd.U = 0 and sd.U
= 0.1 the coverage probability of the naive approach is equal to the benchmark
estimation. In the case of sd.U = 0.4 and sd.U = 0.8 the naive estimation shows
the lowest coverage probability with 92.4% and 76.7.%. For the naive estimation
holds that with increasing error variance the coverage probability is decreasing. The
MSE for sd.U = 0, sd.U = 0.1 and sd.U = 0.4 is nearly the same for all four
approaches. For sd.U = 0.8 the corrected estimation and regression calibration
have a three and two times higher MSE than the benchmark estimation, respectively.
The naive estimation shows a higher MSE than the benchmark estimator, but a
lower MSE compared to the corrected estimation and regression calibration. The
expected failure times are (almost) the same for all approaches considering sd.U =
0 and sd.U = 0.1, respectively. In the case of sd.U = 0.4 and sd.U = 0.8 the
expected failure times are comparable for the benchmark and corrected estimators.
$\widehat{\mathbb{E}(T)}$ of the naive and regression calibration estimators show higher values.

These described tendencies are similar for $\hat{\tau}$ (see Table C.7). Noticeable differences
are: $sd(\hat{\tau})$ is (almost) equal for the benchmark, naive and regression calibration
within each value of the error standard deviation. For no measurement error,
sd.U = 0.1 and sd.U = 0.4, $sd(\hat{\tau})$ of the corrected estimation is equal to the

other approaches. For sd.U = 0.8 it is higher in comparison to the remaining approaches. The coverage probability for the naive estimation is equal to the regression calibration. $\widehat{MSE}$ is rather low for all approaches and sd.Us. The number of failed optimizations is zero, besides for the corrected estimator with sd.U = 0.8. Here, in only 1 of 1000 cases the optimization has failed.

Considering the sample size 500 and 1000 (see Table C.8 and C.9), the tendencies are the same as for 100. All in all, the sample and mean standard deviation as well as the MSE are smaller, whereby these quantities of the corrected estimator move closer to the benchmark estimation. In addition, it can be seen that the coverage probability decreases for the naive estimator and increases for the corrected estimator, so that it becomes closer to the coverage probability of the benchmark estimation and in some parts is higher than for the regression calibration. No failure of optimization is observed for sample size 500 and 1000.

The results for the amount of censoring equal to 35% and 65% are similar to those described above, this means that the estimation accuracy for $\hat{\beta}_V$ is comparable. The difference here is that the estimation of τ is more close to tau.true and is almost equal for the different approaches and error standard deviations. The algorithm does not converge 4 times for 35% and 8 times for 65%, again for the corrected approach and sd.U = 0.8.

The results for $V \sim Unif(0, \sqrt{12})$ are comparable to those with $V \sim N(0, 1)$ as described above (cf. Appendix C.1.4).

The constellation beta.true = -0.2 and tau.true = 0.5 of the simulation grid perform in the same way (see CD, attached to the appendix). The estimation of β_V is comparable for the benchmark, corrected estimation and regression calibration. For the naive estimation the effect is attenuated for increasing error standard deviation. The estimation of τ is closer to tau.true and is almost equal for the different approaches and error standard deviations. In addition, only a few problems with optimization are observed and no outliers are generated.

Conclusion

The performance of the different approaches does not differ fundamentally for sd.U = 0.1 and no measurement error (sd.U = 0). This suggests that for a low measurement error the estimation is not noticeable biased. For sd.U = 0.4 and sd.U = 0.8 the estimation of β_V for the corrected estimation and regression calibration is comparable to the benchmark estimation. The naive estimation

results in biased estimation. The estimation accuracy of $\hat{\tau}$ differs for an increasing
and decreasing hazard rate. For an increasing hazard rate (tau.true = -0.3)
the corrected estimation is comparable to the benchmark estimation. The naive
estimator and the regression calibration are shifted downwards. For a decreasing
hazard rate (tau.true = 0.5) the corrected and benchmark estimation as well as
the regression calibration behave in similar way. The naive estimator results for
some constellations in biased estimation, for other the naive estimation behaves in
an equal way to the other approaches. For an increasing hazard rate the corrected
estimation is in mean better than the naive estimation and the regression calibration,
but with higher variance (bias-variance-trade-off). For a decreasing hazard rate, the
corrected estimation and regression calibration result in comparable estimations.
The sample size influences the variance and the MSE of the estimators. The lager
the sample size, the smaller the variance and the MSE. In total, the amount of
censoring does not seem to influence the estimation accuracy. Problems arise in
the optimization algorithm for the corrected estimation mainly for sample size 100
and sd.U = 0.8 and especially for a censoring amount of 65%. In addition, for
$\tau = -0.3$ more problems with convergence of the optimization algorithm arise.
The results for the different distributions of the true covariate ($V \sim N(0,1)$ and
$V \sim Unif(0, \sqrt{12})$) does not differ fundamentally.

4.1.2. Check the fit Function - W and F

In the thesis the corrected log-likelihood is extended to error-free covariables. To
analyse, if the correction for measurement error is only conducted for the error-
prone covariables and not for the error-free covariables the procedure above is
extended to $A_i = (W_i, F_i)'$. Thus, the data set consists of the censored failure
times and two covariates, one error-free and one error-prone variable. The steps to
generate random numbers in R are the same as in the section before. In addition, an
error-free covariable F_i is generated with $F_i \sim N(0,1)$ (F <-rnorm(size,0,1)). To
generate the failure times a beta.V.true and beta.F.true have to be considered.
One obtains for T_i:

$$T_i = [-log(D_i) \cdot exp((\beta_V' V_i + \beta_F' F_i)/exp(\tau))]^{exp(\tau)} \text{ with } D_i \sim Unif(0,1).$$

The simulation grid is given in Table 4.2. Again a negative and positive value for
beta.V.true and beta.F.true are considered in combination with an increasing
and decreasing hazard rate.

size	sd.U	beta.V.true	beta.F.true	tau.true	prob.cens
100	0	-0.3	-0.1	0.4	0%
500	0.1				35%
1000	0.4				65%
	0.8	-0.3	0.2	0.4	0%
					35%
					65%
		-0.3	-0.1	-0.5	0%
					35%
					65%
		-0.3	0.2	-0.5	0%
					35%
					65%
		0.6	-0.1	0.4	0%
					35%
					65%
		0.6	0.2	0.4	0%
					35%
					65%
		0.6	-0.1	-0.5	0%
					35%
					65%
		0.6	0.2	-0.5	0%
					35%
					65%

Table 4.2.: Simulation grid for *Check the fit Function* with $\tilde{Y} \sim W + F$ and monte.carlo $= 1000$

Results

The results for beta.V.true $= 0.6$, beta.F.true $= $ -0.1, tau.true $= $ -0.5 and prob.cens $= 0\%$ are presented in detail in Appendix C.2.1 for the normally distributed true covariate and for the uniformly distributed covariate in Appendix C.2.2. Starting with V_i normally distributed: The boxplots for $\hat{\beta}_V$, $\hat{\beta}_F$ and $\hat{\tau}$ are depicted in Figure C.25 – C.33 for sample size 100, 500 and 1000. The estimates of β_V with sd.U $= 0$ are equal for all sample sizes, respectively, and the sample median is equal to beta.V.true. For the remaining sd.Us the sample median of the regression calibration and corrected estimator is similar in comparison to the benchmark estimator. For sd.U $= 0.4$ and sd.U $= 0.8$ the range of variation is larger for the corrected estimation and regression calibration. For the naive estimator it can be observed that the larger sd.U and the sample size are, the larger is the attenuation of the true effect. The sample median of $\hat{\beta}_F$ is (almost) equal to beta.F.true for all approaches, all sd.Us and all sample sizes (see Figure C.26, C.29 and C.32). The variation of the naive estimation, regression calibration and corrected estimation is nearly the same, only for sd.U = 0.8 the range is always larger for the corrected estimator. The sample median of $\hat{\tau}$ for sd.U = 0 and sd.U = 0.1 is nearly the same for all approaches, respectively (see Figure C.27, C.30 and C.33). For sample size 100 the effect is overestimated, but for increasing sample size the sample median moves closer to tau.true. For sd.U = 0.4 and sd.U = 0.8 the sample median of the corrected estimators are almost equal to the benchmark estimator, but the variation range is higher. The naive and regression calibration estimates of τ are shifted upwards. Again, the larger the sample size and sd.U are, the larger is the attenuation of the true effect. The summary tables for sample size 100, 500 and 1000 are shown in Table C.13 – C.18. $\hat{\beta}_V$ and $\hat{\beta}_F$ are summarized in one table. The results for $\hat{\tau}$ are shown separately. The accuracy of $\hat{\beta}_V$ is similar to the results of the model with only W as a covariable (see Section 4.1.1). Again, for all approaches and sample sizes, the median and the mean of $\hat{\beta}_V$ are nearly the same, respectively, which is a sign of no outliers. The larger the sample size is, the closer these two quantities move together. $\overline{sd(\hat{\beta}_V)}$ is smaller than $sd(\hat{\beta}_V)$, especially for the corrected estimator. For an increasing sample size this differences are overcome and the values move closer together. For sd.U = 0 and sd.U = 0.1 the values of $sd(\hat{\beta}_V)$ are (almost) equal for the different approaches. For sd.U = 0.4 and sd.U = 0.8 the sample standard deviation of the regression calibration and the corrected estimation is larger in comparison to the benchmark estimation, whereby the corrected estimation shows larger values than the regression calibration. This difference is higher for larger error standard deviation. Noticeable is that the naive estimator shows a smaller standard deviation than the regression calibration and corrected estimators. For sample size 100 the coverage probability (% ∈ CI) of the corrected estimators turns out to be smaller than for the benchmark estimation. The benchmark estimation shows a coverage probability of around 94% and the corrected estimation around 92%. For sd.U = 0.8 the corrected estimation is larger, this could be due to the higher standard deviation of the corrected estimation, which leads to an expanded range of the confidence intervals. The coverage probability of the regression calibration is comparable to the benchmark estimation. Only for sd.U = 0.8 it is a little lower. For sd.U = 0 and sd.U = 0.1 the coverage probability of the naive approach is equal to the benchmark estimation. In the case of sd.U = 0.4 and sd.U = 0.8 the naive estimation shows the lowest coverage probability (69.6% and 3.2%). For the naive estimation holds that with increasing error variance the coverage probability is decreasing, for sample size 500 to 15.1% and 0% and for sample size 1000 to 1.1% and 0%. For increasing sample size the coverage probability of the corrected estimator moves closer to the benchmark estimation and to 95%, which is a sign that the assumption of the normal distribution is justified. For the regression calibration it is still lower compared to the benchmark estimation for sd.U = 0.8. In the case of sd.U = 0.1 the MSE is equal for all approaches and is equal to the one for sd.U = 0. For sample size 100 the MSE of sd.U = 0.4 and sd.U = 0.8 is the highest for the naive estimation. For the corrected estimator and regression calibration it is higher than for the benchmark estimation. This difference becomes less for increasing sample size.

For $\hat{\beta}_F$ no attenuation is observed for increasing variance of the measurement error. $\hat{\beta}_F$ shows higher standard deviation for the naive estimation, regression calibration and corrected estimation in comparison to the benchmark estimation. For sd.U = 0.4 the standard deviations for the naive estimation, regression calibration and the corrected estimation are closer together, than for sd.U = 0.8. Here, the corrected estimator always has the highest standard deviation. Considering sample size 100 the coverage probability for sd.U = 0 and sd.U = 0.1, the naive estimation and regression calibration show (almost) equal coverage probabilities. The corrected estimator lies a little under the remaining approaches. For sd.U = 0.4 and sd.U = 0.8 the naive and the corrected estimation as well as the regression calibration have a lower coverage probability compared to the benchmark estimator. For increasing sample size the coverage probability for $\hat{\beta}_F$ increases and the corrected estimation moves closer to the benchmark estimator. All in all, the MSE is rather small and comparable for all approaches and sd.Us. For sample size 100 and 500 as well as sd.U = 0.4 and sd.U = 0.8 the MSE of the corrected estimator is two times larger than the benchmark estimation. The estimated expected failure time is the same in the case of sd.U = 0 and sd.U = 0.1 for all approaches and sample sizes, respectively. For sd.U = 0.4 and sd.U = 0.8 the corrected expected failure time is always equal or quite close to the benchmark expected failure time. The naive estimation and regression calibration differs, for sd.U = 0.8 more than for sd.U = 0.4 and tends to overestimate $\widehat{\mathbb{E}(T)}$.

For $\hat{\tau}$ the behaviour of the corrected estimation is nearly the same as for $\hat{\beta}_V$. Noticeable difference are: The regression calibration performs in a comparable way to the naive estimation considering the sample mean and median as well as the standard deviation, the coverage probability and the MSE. This means that the effect of the regression calibration approach is also attenuated. For sd.U = 0.8 the corrected estimation failed the optimization 362 times out of 500 repetitions for sample size 100 and 26 times for sample size 500. For sample size 1000 and for the remaining repetitions no problems occurred.

All in all, the standard deviation for the estimation and the MSE decrease for increasing sample size. The results do not differ basically for the different amounts of censorship. Only the number of failed optimizations for the corrected approach increases and for 65% censorship this problem arises also for the other approaches. In addition, for censorship of 35% and 65% outliers are generated for all sample sizes and for all approaches. It can be observed that in the case of an outlier for $\hat{\beta}_V$, outliers are also generated for $\hat{\beta}_F$ and $\hat{\tau}$. This means that the estimation goes wrong in total.

Again, the results for $V \sim Unif(0, \sqrt{12})$ do not differ from those for $V \sim N(0,1)$ as described above (cf. Appendix C.2.2).

For the remaining cells of the simulation grid it is observed that all cells with tau.true = -0.5 behave in a similar way as described above with regard to the estimation accuracy and to failure of optimizations as well as to the generation of outliers. All cells with tau.true = 0.4 result in similar estimations. The estimation accuracy for $\hat{\beta}_V$ and $\hat{\beta}_F$ is similar to those with tau.true = -0.5. The estimation of τ differs. Here, the attenuation of the true effect for the naive estimator and regression calibration is less presented or is not given. Only optimization problems occur for sample size 100 with sd.U = 0.8 and no outliers are generated.

The results for $V \sim Unif(0, \sqrt{12})$ do not differ from those for $V \sim N(0,1)$. Again the same tendencies are observed for the cells with tau.true = 0.4 and tau.true = -0.5, respectively.

Conclusion

The results for sd.U = 0 are equal for the different approaches and the sample median is equal to the true parameter value. This means that in the absence of measurement error all approaches indeed are the same. For sd.U = 0.1, sd.U = 0.4 and sd.U = 0.8 the sample median of the corrected estimation and regression calibration of β_V is in most of the cases equal to the one of the benchmark estimation,

but the variance is higher. The naive estimators are attenuated downwards, for
sd.U = 0.8 stronger than for sd.U = 0.4 and sd.U = 0.1. For $\hat{\beta}_F$ the median for
all approaches, all sd.Us and all sample sizes are (almost) equal to beta.F.true.
Including an error-free covariable in the corrected log-likelihood works out well. For
$\hat{\tau}$ the median for sd.U = 0 and sd.U = 0.1 are nearly the same. The larger the
sample size is, the closer the sample median is equal to tau.true. For sd.U = 0.4
and sd.U = 0.8 the estimation accuracy for the cells with tau.true = 0.4 and
tau.true = -0.5 does not differ in the case of $\hat{\beta}_V$ and $\hat{\beta}_F$, but for the estimation
of τ. In the case of tau.true = -0.5 the corrected estimation is comparable to
the benchmark estimation, but with a higher variance. The naive estimator and
regression calibration are attenuated. The larger the error standard deviation is,
the larger is the attenuation of the effect. In the case of tau.true = 0.4 the
regression calibration and corrected estimation behave in a similar way and are
comparable to the benchmark estimation. The effect of the naive estimation is
shifted. Problems arise in the optimization algorithm for the corrected estimation.
These problems arise mainly for sample size 100 with sd.U = 0.8 and for tau.true
= -0.5 and more seriously for an amount of censoring of 65%. For tau.true =
0.4 no outliers are generated. In total, the amount of censoring does not seem to
influence the estimation accuracy, only on the amount of failed optimizations. The
sample size influences the variance and the MSE of the estimators. The lager the
sample size is, the smaller the variance and MSE are. The results for the different
distributions ($V \sim N(0,1)$ and $V \sim Unif(0, \sqrt{12})$) of the true covariate do not
differ fundamentally.

4.2. Structural Changes

In the first part of the simulation study, it was shown that for V_i normally distributed and V_i uniformly distributed the performance does not differ fundamentally.
Therefore, only V_i normally distributed is considered. Similarly, it was shown that
the inclusion of an error-free covariable F_i in the optimization works out well. Thus,
here only W_i is considered as a covariable.

The question of interest is, if the new implemented estimation technique identifies
parameter instability (structural change) within the MOB algorithm. As a quality
criterion the proportion of the true detected structural changes is taken, which
is compared to the benchmark estimation, naive estimation and the regression
calibration. In addition, the estimation accuracy of the different approaches are

considered.

4.2.1. Structural Changes - single

At first one single structural change should be detected, as shown in Figure 4.1. Under the assumption of an additive measurement error model with homoscedastic normal errors (see Section 2.1.1), a data set is simulated, which integrates the underlying tree structure in the data generating process. Only one covariate, which is subject to measurement error and one binary partitioning variable are considered. Thus, the data set consists of the failure times and the censoring indicator as well as the error-prone covariate and the partitioning variable. Here, it is limited to one type of partitioning variables. In R the following steps are conducted to generate the random numbers (cf. Section 4.1.1):

1. The covariable for a fixed value of σ_U^2 and partitioning variable:

   - True covariable: $V_i \sim N(0,1)$ (V <-rnorm(size,0,1))
   - Measurement error: $U_i \sim N(0,\sigma_U^2)$ (U <-rnorm(size,0,sd.U))
   - $\rightarrow W_i = V_i + U_i$
   - Partitioning variable Z_{1_i}, where $Z_{1_i} \in \{0,1\}$ (Z1 <- runif(size, min = 0, max = 1), Z1[Z1 < 0.5] <- 0 and Z1[Z1 >= 0.5] <- 1)

2. The censored failure times $\tilde{Y}_i = (min(T_i, C_i), \delta_i)$:

   - Failure time: The MOB algorithm should detect one split point in Z_1, this means for T_i:

   $$T_i = \begin{cases} [-log(D_i) \cdot exp(\beta_1' V_i / exp(\tau_1))]^{exp(\tau_1)} & , \text{if } Z_{1_i} = 0 \\ [-log(D_i) \cdot exp(\beta_2' V_i / exp(\tau_2))]^{exp(\tau_2)} & , \text{if } Z_{1_i} = 1 \end{cases}$$

   - Censoring time: Since C_i is independent of $\beta_V' V_i$, the censoring variable is generated from an uniform distribution. C <- runif(size, min = 0, max = b.cens), where b.cens is chosen in such a way that the proportion of censoring is controlled.
   - $\rightarrow \delta_i = 0$, if $T_i > C_i$ (censored) and $\delta_i = 1$, if $T_i \leq C_i$ (event)
   - $\rightarrow \tilde{Y}_i = (min(T_i, C_i), \delta_i)$

The simulated data set is used to fit the MOB. The different approaches are computed in R in the following way

- Benchmark estimation:
  ```
  mob(Surv(time,status) ~ V | Z1, data = data, control = ctrl,
  model = survReg)
  ```

- Naive estimation:
  ```
  mob(Surv(time,status) ~ W | Z1, data = data, control = ctrl,
  model = survReg)
  ```

- Regression calibration:
  ```
  mob(Surv(time,status) ~ W.reg.calib | Z1, data = data,
  control = ctrl, model = survReg),
  ```
  where W. reg.calib are the conditional expectations, computed as in Equation (2.10).

- Corrected estimation:
  ```
  mob(Surv(time,status) ~ W | Z1, data = data, control = ctrl,
  model = SurvRegcorr, error.var = "W", sd.U = sd.U)
  ```

where the control parameter crtl is set to

```
mob_control(objfun = function(object){-as.vector(logLik(object))}).
```

This means that the control parameters of the MOB algorithm are set to the default values, besides the objfun is set to the negative log-likelihood (cf. Section 3.2). The different approaches are compared with respect to the ability to detect the underlying structural change. Therefore, a variable count.mob is introduced, which counts the number of true detected tree structures for each approach, respectively. The resulting mob object includes detailed information about the tree structure. With if-queries the true tree structure is checked as well as the split point. The resulting tree must be of the structure that the left and right daughter node from the first node are terminal nodes and the split point is equal to 0. If the first node is already the terminal node, the true underlying tree structure is not detected and the variable count.mob remains constant.

In Table 4.3 the simulation grid is shown. Four different constellations are checked. At first $\beta_1 = \beta_2$ and $\tau_1 = \tau_2$, here the effect of the covariate V on the response variable is independent of the partitioning variable Z_1, this means that no parameter

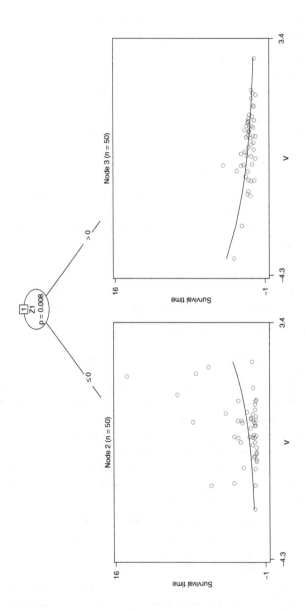

Figure 4.1.: MOB estimated via the corrected approach with beta.1.true = 0.6, beta.2.true = -0.2, tau.1.true = 0.5, tau.2.true = -0.4, prob.cens = 35%, $V \sim N(0,1)$, size = 1000 and sd.U = 0.4

size	sd.U	beta.1.true	beta.2.true	tau.1.true	tau.2.true	prob.cens
100	0	0.3	0.3	0.5	0.5	0%
500	0.1					35%
1000	0.4					65%
	0.8	0.6	-0.2	0.5	0.5	0%
						35%
						65%
		0.3	0.3	0.5	-0.4	0%
						35%
						65%
		0.6	-0.2	0.5	-0.4	0%
						35%
						65%

Table 4.3.: Simulation grid for *Structural Changes* with $\tilde{Y} \sim W \mid Z_1$ and monte.carlo = 500

instability exits. The false discovery rate is examined, this means that the MOB algorithm detects a parameter instability, even though there is no one. This corresponds to the Type-I-error. Moreover, three different constellations are analysed: $\beta_1 \neq \beta_2$ and $\tau_1 = \tau_2$, $\beta_1 = \beta_2$ and $\tau_1 \neq \tau_2$ as well as $\beta_1 \neq \beta_2$ and $\tau_1 \neq \tau_2$.

The sample size is set to 100, 500, 1000. Note, this means around half sample size per terminal node. The error standard deviation as well as the amount of censorship is chosen as above. The procedure is repeated 500 times. For some constellations of the simulation grid and simulated data the MOB algorithm fails to fit the model due to convergence problems. In this case the MOB is counted as a not detected true tree structure, here the variable count.mob remain constant. In addition, a variable count.NA is introduced, it counts the number of failed MOB algorithm. For every true detected tree the parameter estimations of the two terminal nodes 2 and 3 are saved (cf. Figure 4.1). The averages and the standard deviation of the resulting parameter estimation (see (4.1) – (4.4)) as well as the coverage probability are computed and only base on those observations, where the MOB algorithm detects the true underlying tree structure, i. e. mc = count.mob. For the corrected MOB algorithm not only the modified file SurvRegcorr.sim.r is included, also the implemented functions for the new object SurvRegcorr are considered in the MOB algorithm, such as estfun.SurvRegcorr(), logLik. SurvRegcorr(), print.SurvRegcorr(), reweight.SurvRegcorr() and weights. SurvRegcorr() as described in Section 3.2.

Results

The results for `beta.1.true` = 0.6, `beta.2.true` = -0.2 , `tau.1.true` = 0.5,
`tau.2.true` = -0.4, `prob.cens` = 35% and $V_i \sim N(0,1)$ are shown in Appendix
4.2.1 and are analysed in detail in the following. In Table C.25, C.28 and C.31 the
results for the detection of structural changes for sample size 100, 500 and 1000 are
shown. The tables include the percentage of true detected trees (%#mob) and the
absolute value (#mob). In addition, the number of not detected true structural
changes (not #mob) and the number of failed optimizations (#NA) are printed,
where #NA specifies the number of how many of the not detected mobs are due
to failure of the optimization. For sample size 500 and 1000 the detection rate
for all approaches and `sd.Us` are 100%. This means that the different approaches
do not differ in the detection of the true underlying tree structure. Considering
sample size 100, for `sd.U` = 0 the percentage for all approaches is equal to 92%.
For `sd.U` = 0.1 the benchmark estimator has with 91.2%, the naive and regression
calibration and the corrected estimation have a smaller rate with 90.6%, 90.6%
and 90.4%, respectively. A similar tendency is observed for `sd.U` = 0.4. For `sd.U`
= 0.8 the benchmark estimation detects in 92.8% of the 500 repetitions the true
tree structure, the naive and regression calibration only in 88.2%. The corrected
estimation detects only 70.2%, but in 82 cases of the not detected structural change
the optimization fails. If one would add these 82 to the 351 detected structural
changes, the proportion would be 86.6%, which is closer to the one of the naive
estimation and regression calibration.

The results of 0% and 65% censoring are comparable for sample size 500 and 1000,
here the detection rate is equal to 100% for 0% censoring and a little less than
100% for 65% censoring. For sample size 100 and 0% censoring the detection rate
varies between 83% and 85%, where the different approaches are comparable within
the different values of `sd.U`. For `sd.U` = 0.8 the corrected estimator shows 54 NAs
and thus only a detection rate of 72%. For 65% censoring the detection rate drops
down to 62% - 63%. For `sd.U` = 0.8 the benchmark estimation shows the highest
detection rate with 64%. The naive approach and regression calibration lie with
56% under it and the corrected estimation shows again 67 NAs and thus only a
detection rate of 42%.

In the two terminal nodes a different τ is included. For `tau.1.true` = 0.5 a
decreasing hazard rate is simulated, which means that the probability for an event
decreases over the time and at the same time the probability to survive increases.

For `tau.2.true` = -0.4 an increasing hazard rate is simulated this means that the probability for an event increases over the time, and thus the probability to survive decreases. These tendencies can also be seen in the resulting plots of the two terminal nodes in Figure 4.1. For terminal node 2 with true underlying τ_1 the estimated median survival curve shows an increasing line. For terminal node 3 with true underlying τ_2 the median survival time is decreasing over the time. The resulting tree for the benchmark and naive estimation as well as for the regression calibration does not differ, except the p-value of the parameter instability test for Z_1.

Furthermore, the resulting parameter estimation in the two terminal nodes is analysed. The boxplots for $\hat{\beta}_1$, $\hat{\beta}_2$, $\hat{\tau}_1$ and $\hat{\tau}_2$ are shown in Figure C.43 – C.46 for sample size 100, in Figure C.47 – C.50 for sample size 500 and in Figure C.51 – C.54 for sample size 1000. The resulting estimation in the two terminal nodes behave in a similar way as for considering the fit functions separately (see Section 4.1.1). Again, for $\hat{\beta}_1$ and $\hat{\beta}_2$ the results of `sd.U` = 0.1 are similar to those with no measurement error. The sample median for all approaches is almost equal to `beta.1.true` and `beta.2.true`, respectively. For `sd.U` = 0.4 and `sd.U` = 0.8 the sample median of the corrected estimation and the regression calibration are comparable to the benchmark estimation, but with a higher variance. The naive estimation is shifted. For increasing sample size the attenuation becomes again more apparent. For sample size 100 and `sd.U` = 0.4 outliers are generated in terminal node 3 for the naive estimation, regression calibration and corrected estimation.

The estimation of τ_1 and τ_2 are comparable for `sd.U` = 0 and `sd.U` = 0.1. The sample median of all approaches lies a little under the true effect. For increasing sample size the sample median moves closer to `tau.1.true` and `tau.2.true`, respectively. For `sd.U` = 0.4 and `sd.U` = 0.8 the performance of the corrected estimators are comparable to the benchmark estimator. The naive approach and the regression calibration behave in a similar way. Here, the effect of `tau.1.true` is overestimated and the effect of `tau.2.true` is shifted downwards. The larger the sample size is, the stronger is the attenuation of $\hat{\tau}_2$.

The summary tables are given in Table C.26 and C.27 for sample size 100, C.29 and C.30 for sample size 500 and C.32 and C.33 for sample size 1000. The output of terminal node 2 including the results of $\hat{\beta}_1$ and $\hat{\tau}_1$ as well as the output of terminal node 3 including the results of $\hat{\beta}_2$ and $\hat{\tau}_2$ are depicted separately. For each parameter the same quantities are shown as described in Equation (4.1) – (4.6) as well as the coverage probability ($\% \in$ CI). All in all, the resulting tables do not differ fundamentally from those, where the performance of the fit functions is analysed separately (see Section 4.1.1). Again, for an increasing sample size the standard deviation and the MSE is decreasing. Noticeable is that the standard deviation of $\hat{\beta}_1$ turns out to be around two times larger than for $\hat{\beta}_2$. For sample size 100 and sd.U = 0.4 the results in terminal node 3 are biased, because of the outliers, which can be seen in the boxplots. The resulting estimations are comparable for 0% and 65% censoring. For 65% a many problems with outliers arise in the case of estimating β_2 and τ_2.

Considering the other simulation cells (see CD, attached to the appendix): For beta.1.true = 0.3, beta.2.true = 0.3 , tau.1.true = 0.5, tau.2.true = 0.5 no structural change is generated. Here, the resulting parameter estimation is not considered, because the resulting tree is not of interest and the average only is based on a few observations. The false discover rate is of interest. The results for the different amounts of censorship do not differ fundamentally. For sample size 100 2% - 4% are falsely detected. Within the different values of the sd.Us the approaches perform in a comparable way. For sample size 500 the false discover rate varies between 2% - 7%, where in the case sd.U = 0.8 the benchmark estimator shows a higher number of falsely detected trees than the other approaches. For sample size 1000 in 4% - 7% of the 500 repetitions a structural change is falsely detected. Within the sd.Us the approaches perform in a comparable way. For no censoring the differences are maximal 3 trees. For an amount of 35% censoring the differences are maximal 4 trees and for 65% maximal 6 trees. For increasing sample size the Type-I-error lies around 5%, which is equal to the significance level of 5% and was determined in mob_control().

The results for beta.1.true = 0.3, beta.2.true = 0.3, tau.1.true = 0.5, tau.2.true = -0.4 are similar to those described above. All in all, the different approaches perform within the individual sd.Us in a comparable way. For sample size 100 and no censoring the proportion of true detected tree structure varies around 80%, except the corrected approaches with sd.U = 0.8. It is only 70.4%, but in 49 cases the MOB algorithm is failed. For 35% censoring the rate lies between 72% and 80%, and again the corrected estimator shows 60 NAs for sd.U = 0.8 and thus shows only a detection rate of 62.6%. For 65% censoring the detection rate drops down to 40% - 50%. For sd.U = 0.8 the corrected estimator fails 51 times and shows a detection rate of only 37.4%. For sample size 500 and 1000 the detection rate is again 100% for 0% and 35% censoring, for 65% it is a little less than 100%. The resulting parameter estimation is comparable to those from described above. Again problems with outliers occur for 65% censoring. For beta.1.true = 0.6, beta.2.true = -0.2, tau.1.true = 0.5, tau.2.true = 0.5 the detection rate is lower than for the other two constellations. It is getting worse for increasing censorship amount. In general it can be seen that the different approaches perform in a similar way within sd.U = 0 and sd.U = 0.1. For sd.U = 0.4 and sd.U = 0.8 the naive estimation, regression calibration and corrected estimation show lower values compared to the benchmark estimation. Due to arising NAs for the corrected estimator in the case of sd.U = 0.8 the corrected estimator lies under the naive and regression calibration approach. For sample size 100 the rate only varies between 12% and 18% and falls down to 7% - 10% for an amount of censoring of 65%. For sample size 500 the detection rate turns out to be higher (90% - 96% for 0% censoring), but with increasing amount of censoring the rate decreases to around 50% for 65% censoring. For sample size 1000 the detection rate moves closer to 100% for 0% and 35% censoring. For 65% censoring it varies from 65% to over 90%. The resulting parameter estimations of β_1 and β_2 are overestimated and of τ_1 and τ_2 are underestimated for sample size 100. This can be traced back to the small amount of detected trees, so that the averages only is based on a small amount of values. For 500 and 1000 the estimation is similar to the estimation described above. Again, the regression calibration and corrected estimation provide similar estimations for β_1 and β_2 compared to the benchmark estimation. The naive estimator is attenuated for sd.U = 0.4 and sd.U = 0.8. For τ_1 the regression calibration and the naive estimation are shifted a little upwards for sd.U = 0.4 and sd.U = 0.8. For $\hat{\tau}_2$ these differences in comparison to the benchmark and corrected estimation cannot be observed, here the four approaches perform in a comparable way.

Conclusion

The larger the sample size is, the more true structural changes are detected. The false detection rate lies around 5%. With increasing amount of censorship the detection rate is getting worse. The results provide evidence that structural changes could be better detected for $\beta_1 = \beta_2$ and $\tau_1 \neq \tau_2$ than for $\beta_1 \neq \beta_2$ and $\tau_1 = \tau_2$. The results of the first constellation are comparable to those where $\beta_1 \neq \beta_2$ and $\tau_1 \neq \tau_2$. This suggests that a difference in τ and accordingly for ν (shape parameter of the Weibull distribution) is easier to detect than a difference in β. For sd.U = 0.8 the corrected estimation has almost always problems with optimization.

Thus the detection rate is lower than for the other approaches. If one would add the number of NAs to the number of detected trees, the resulting proportion is close to the remaining approaches. For the resulting parameter estimation, similar results can be observed as for the separated consideration of the fit functions in Section 4.1.1. In general, for the estimation of β_1 and β_2 the regression calibration and the corrected estimator are equal to the benchmark estimation, respectively. The naive estimator is shifted upwards or downwards from sd.U = 0.4. For the estimation of τ_1 and τ_2 the estimation for sd.U = 0, sd.U = 0.1 and sd.U = 0.4 are almost the same for the four different approaches. For sd.U = 0.8 the corrected estimation is equal to the benchmark. The regression calibration and naive estimation are shifted upwards or downwards. The larger the sample size, the large the attenuation. For sd.U = 0.1 the standard deviation of the corrected estimator is almost the same as for the other approaches. For sd.U = 0.4 and sd.U = 0.8 the standard deviations are larger than for the benchmark estimation, and are larger than for the naive estimation and the regression calibration, whereas the regression calibration standard deviation often lies close to the corrected one. Here, again the variance-bias-trade-off problem occurs.

4.2.2. Structural Changes - multi

The procedure is extended to more than one structural change. Here, three terminal nodes should be detected (cf. Figure 4.2). The simulated data set consists of the censored failure times, one covariate and two partitioning variables. The steps to generate random numbers in R are the same as above (see Section 4.2.1). In addition, a continuous partitioning variable Z_2 is generated with $Z_2 \sim Unif(0,1)$ (Z2 <- runif(size,0,1)). To simulate the failure times a beta.1.true, beta.2.true and beta.3.true as well as tau.1.true, tau.2.true and tau.3.true have to be considered. For T_i one obtains:

$$T_i = \begin{cases} [-log(D_i) \cdot exp(\beta_1' V_i/exp(\tau_1))]^{exp(\tau_1)} & \text{, if } Z_{1_i} = 0 \\ [-log(D_i) \cdot exp(\beta_2' V_i/exp(\tau_2))]^{exp(\tau_2)} & \text{, if } Z_{1_i} = 1 \text{ and } Z_{2_i} \geq 0.5 \\ [-log(D_i) \cdot exp(\beta_3' V_i/exp(\tau_3))]^{exp(\tau_3)} & \text{, if } Z_{1_i} = 1 \text{ and } Z_{2_i} < 0.5. \end{cases} \quad (4.7)$$

The simulation grid is given in Table 4.4. As in Section 4.2.1 three different constellations are analysed: $\beta_1 \neq \beta_2 \neq \beta_3$ and $\tau_1 = \tau_2 = \tau_3$, $\beta_1 = \beta_2 = \beta_3$ and $\tau_1 \neq \tau_2 \neq \tau_3$ as well as $\beta_1 \neq \beta_2 \neq \beta_3$ and $\tau_1 \neq \tau_2 \neq \tau_3$. No structural change does

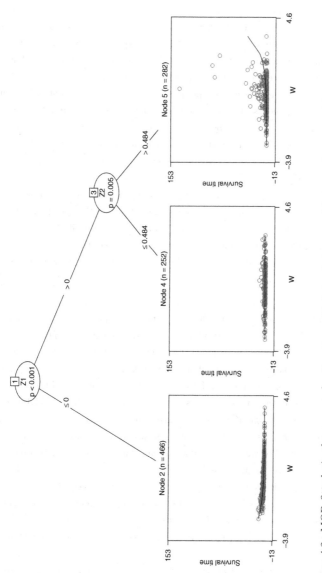

Figure 4.2.: MOB fitted via the corrected estimation with beta.1.true $= -0.9$, beta.2.true $= 0.2$, beta.3.true $= 1.1$, tau.1.true $= -1$, tau.2.true $= 0.1$, tau.3.true $= 0.9$, prob.cens $= 0\%$, $V \sim N(0, 1)$, size $= 1000$ and sd.U $= 0.4$

not make sense here, because very few true tree structures are detected.

Again, a variable count.mob and a variable count.NA are introduced to count the number of detected true tree structures and the number of failed optimizations, respectively. The true tree structure is characterized as follows: The first node is split for the partitioning variable Z_1 with the split point equal to zero. The left daughter node is a terminal node. The right daughter node is split further for the partitioning variable Z_2 with split point around 0.5. The two resulting daughter nodes are terminal nodes. These characteristics of the tree are saved in the resulting mob object and can be checked by if-queries. The averages and standard deviations of the resulting parameter estimates are not computed, because these calculations would only base on a few observations. The true detected trees are saved as a mob object, respectively.

As noted in Section 3.2 a continuous partitioning variable the new implemented fit function SurvRegcorr@fit() takes a long time to find the split point. For Z_2 (size - 1) possible cut points, if no ties are available, are obtained. This means that for an increasing sample size the running time increases. For the binary partitioning variable Z_1 this problem does not occur, because here only one cut point is possible.

Results

In Appendix C.4 the summary tables are depicted for all constellations in Table 4.4. The tables include the percentage of true detected trees (%#mob) and the absolute value (#mob). In addition, the number of not detected true structural changes (not #mob) and the number of failed optimizations (#NA) are printed, where #NA specifies the number of how many of the not detected MOBs are due to failure of the optimization. The results for the different values of sd.U and for sample size 100, 500 and 1000 are summarized in one table. For sample size 100 only 0 - 6 true trees are detected. The problem here is that for the left terminal node around 50 observations are allocated and for the remaining two terminal nodes only 25 observations per node are left. In most of the cases it holds that the larger the sample size is, the larger the number of detected trees. However, still the rate is very low, the maximum lies at 19 trees out of 500 repetitions that is only 3.8%. In several test runs it was observed that mainly only the single tree structure was detected with split point in Z_1, which is not equal to the true underlying tree structure.

Again problems with the optimization arise for the corrected approach, mainly for

size	sd.U	beta.1.true	beta.2.true	beta.3.true	tau.1.true	tau.2.true	tau.3.true	prob.cens
100	0	-0.9	0.2	1.1	0.5	0.5	0.5	0%
500	0.1							35%
1000	0.4							65%
	0.8	0.4	0.4	0.4	-1	0.1	0.9	0%
								35%
								65%
		-0.9	0.2	1.1	-1	0.1	0.9	0%
								35%
								65%

Table 4.4.: Simulation grid for *Structural Changes* with $\bar{Y} \sim W \mid Z_1 + Z_2$ and monte.carlo = 500

sd.U = 0.8. For some constellations of the simulation grid this problem arises for lower error standard deviations as well.

The naive estimation and regression calibration show equal detection rates. The corrected estimation performs in different ways. For some constellations it shows an equal detection rate to the naive estimation and regression calibration as well as to the benchmark estimation. For other constellations the corrected estimation shows a lower detection rate, especially for sd.U = 0.4 and sd.U = 0.8, which could be due to the upcoming problems with the optimization. The benchmark estimation behaves also in a heterogeneous way. For some constellation it shows a higher detection rate in other a lower compared to the remaining approaches. However, the results for sd.U = 0 within each sample size are equal, so that in the absence of measurement error all approaches do the same, as it should be. For sd.U = 0.1 the naive and corrected estimator as well as the regression calibration yield to the same detection rate, which is comparable to the benchmark estimation. With increasing amount of censoring, the number of detected trees decrease.

On the basis of one example the resulting tree with its parameter estimation is described in the following. For beta.1.true = -0.9, beta.2.true = 0.2, beta.3.true = 1.1, tau.1.true = -1, tau.2.true = 0.1, tau.3.true = 0.9, prob.cens = 0% and size = 1000 the correct detected tree is shown in Figure 4.2. This resulting tree is obtained by the corrected estimation with sd.U = 0.4. In the three terminal nodes a different τ is included. For tau.1.true = -1 an increasing hazard rate is simulated, which means that the probability for an event increases over the time and at the same time the probability to survive decreases. For tau.2.true = 0.1 and tau.3.true = 0.9 a decreasing hazard rate is simulated, where the decrement for tau.2.true = 0.1 is lower than for tau.3.true = 0.9. The probability for an event decreases over the time, and thus the probability to survive increases. These tendencies can also be seen in the resulting plots of the three terminal nodes in Figure 4.2. For terminal node 2 with true underlying τ_1 the estimated median survival curve shows a slightly decreasing line. For terminal node 4 with true underlying τ_2 the median survival time is rather constant over the time and for terminal node 5 with true underlying τ_3 the survival time is increasing over the time. The resulting tree for the benchmark and naive estimation as well as for the regression calibration does not differ, except the p-value of the parameter instability test for Z_2, which is equal to 0.012 for the benchmark estimation and 0.004 for the naive estimation and regression calibration. The resulting parameter estimation in the three terminal nodes is different for the approaches, which is printed in Appendix C.4.1. The results for terminal node 2 is marked with $'2'$, for terminal node 4 with $'4'$ and for terminal node 5 with $'5'$. For all terminal nodes the estimators of β are attenuated for the naive estimation in comparison to the benchmark estimation. The estimation of τ is also attenuated for terminal node 2, for terminal node 4 and 5 the resulting estimation is close to the benchmark estimation. The regression calibration result in similar estimations compared to the benchmark estimation, except $\hat{\tau}_1$, here the estimated effect is smaller. The results of the corrected estimator are comparable to the benchmark estimation.

It is not possible to make a statement regarding the variance of the resulting estimation and if the resulting estimation is in mean close to the true estimation as well as to the effect of the different amounts of censoring on the parameter estimation.

At seeing through the single results, the resulting estimations for sample size 100 deviate strongly from the true parameter values. For increasing sample size the estimation moves closer to the true values, but there are still outliers left. In general, the estimation of terminal node 2 turns out to be closer to the true values, but here the sample size is twice of the other two terminal nodes. For increasing error variance the naive estimation is attenuated for all sample sizes.

Conclusion

The detection rate for the true underlying tree structure is rather low. The different approaches perform in a comparable way, therefore this problem cannot be traced back to the new implemented corrected MOB algorithm. Again, for sd.U = 0.8 the corrected estimation has problems with optimization.

However, considering the model summaries of the corrected parameter estimation suggests that the parameter estimation is comparable to the benchmark estimation as well as is close to the true values, except for sample size 100. The regression calibration results in similar estimation. Again, the naive estimation shows biased parameter estimation. These observations were only made at seeing through the single results, therefore further investigations have to be carried out.

4.3. One Global Model Fit vs. MOB

The researcher can decide between one global model fit and a partitioned model with respect to some chosen partitioning variables. Here, the partitioned Weibull

model fitted via the MOB algorithm and the global Weibull model fitted via the
survreg() function are compared. The question of interest is, if there is a profit
in partitioning the data set with respect to some partitioning variables. Again the
benchmark estmation, naive estimation and corrected estimation as well as the
regression calibration are considered.

For the MOB a single structural change as in Figure 4.1 is assumed. The model
equation is specified as follows:

$$\tilde{Y} \sim W|Z_1, \tag{4.8}$$

where $\tilde{Y}$ denotes the censored survival times, W the error-prone covariable and Z_1
the partitioning variable. The equivalence for the global model is

$$\tilde{Y} \sim W + Z_1 + W \cdot Z_1. \tag{4.9}$$

For the global model the problem arises that the error-prone variable is also included
in the interaction term. A corrected log-likelihood has to be derived, which includes
an adjustment for the main effect of the error-prone variable but also for the
effect of the interaction term. In Appendix B.6 such a corrected log-likelihood is
derived for the Weibull model, which fulfils the condition (2.13). Furthermore, the
corrected score functions are derived from the corrected log-likelihood for normal
homoscedastic errors (see Equation (B.18), (B.19) and (B.20)). These results are
integrated in the SurvRegcorr@fit() function and are saved in a function called
SurvRegcorrInter@fit(). A new object SurvRegcorrInter of class StatModel
is generated with modified fit function SurvRegcorrInter@fit() including the
correction for measurement errors for the main and interaction effect. The returned
object is of class SurvRegcorr and survreg, so that the additionally implemented
functions such as logLik.SurvRegcorr() can be allocated to this object (see
Section 3.2). The new object is saved in SurvRegcorr.sim.inter.r, which also
includes an absorption of error warnings in the case of a failed optimization.
For the corrected MOB the modified SurvRegcorr@fit(), which is located in
SurvRegcorr.sim.r is used again. It absorbs the error warnings in the case of a
failed optimization.

A correction for interaction terms with error-prone covariables is not implemented
generally, it was only adopted especially for the given model equation from Equation
(4.9). The integration of a corrected log-likelihood in the MOB algorithm, which

can also include a correction for interaction terms with error-prone covariables, is not considered here. The reason is that the general concept of the MOB includes an automated interaction detection as well as an automated variable selection. Thus, the intuitively procedure would be to pass a model equation with main effects of the covariates to the MOB algorithm and to pass further covariates as partitioning variables. However, the example from the model of Equation (4.9) shows that it is possible to include an adjustment for interaction terms with error-prone variables into the corrected log-likelihood as well as into the MOB algorithm and that is an interesting issue for further research.

The steps for the generation of random numbers in R are the same as in Section 4.2.1. Thus, the data set consists of the failure times and the censoring indicator as well as the error-prone covariate and the partitioning variable. The simulation grid is equal to the one of Table 4.3, but without any structural change, which does not apply here, because the MOB should be compared to the global model.

The partitioned and global model are compared via the prediction accuracy. The prediction error for each model should be considered, but the prediction of censored observations is not intuitive. Therefore, a robust alternative to the Schemper-Henderson estimator (Schemper and Henderson, 2000) is considered, which was derived by Schmid et al. (2011) and quantifies the absolute distance between predicted and observed survival functions and is robust against misspecification of the survival model in the case of the random censoring assumption. The idea of this measure is to consider the time-dependent mean absolute deviation between the survival functions of the prediction model and the true survival states of the observations in the data set and is based on the fundamental principle that the prediction rules is evaluated on independent training and test data (Schmid et al., 2011). The integrated area under the time-dependent prediction error curve is used as a measure of the prediction error and is standardized to the interval [0,1]. In the package survAUC (Potapov et al., 2011) a function predErr() is available to compute this robust measure of prediction error in R. For the calculation of the prediction error the simulated data is split into an independent training data set train.data and a test data set test.data. The partition is done randomly by the sample() function. On the basis of the training data the MOB and the global model is fitted as follows:

- Benchmark estimation:
  ```
  mob(Surv(time,status) ~ V | Z1 , data = train.data, control =
  ctrl, model = survReg)
  ```

`survreg(Surv(time,status)` $\sim$ `V + Z1 + interV, data = train.data)`,
where `interV` is the product of `V` and `Z1`.

- Naive estimation:
  `mob(Surv(time,status)` $\sim$ `W | Z1 , data = train.data, control =`
  `ctrl, model = survReg)`
  `survreg(Surv(time,status)` $\sim$ `W + Z1 + interW, data = train.data)`,
  where `interW` is the product of `W` and `Z1`.

- Regression calibration:
  `mob(Surv(time,status)` $\sim$ `W.reg.calib | Z1 , data = train.data,`
  `control = ctrl, model = survReg)`
  `survreg(Surv(time,status)` $\sim$ `W.reg.calib + Z1 +`
  `interW.reg.calib, data = train.data)`,
  where `interW.reg.calib` is the product of `W.reg.calib` and `Z1`.
  `W.reg.calib` are the conditional expectations, computed as in Equation
  (2.10).

- Corrected estimation:
  `mob(Surv(time,status)` $\sim$ `W | Z1, data = train.data, control =`
  `ctrl, model = SurvRegcorr, error.var = c("W"), sd.U = sd.U)`
  `SurvRegcorrInter@fit(object, weights = NULL, error.var =`
  `error.vars, sd.U = sd.error.vars)`,
  with `object = Surv(time,status)`$\sim$ `W + Z1 + interW, error.vars =`
  `c("W", "interW")` and `sd.error.vars = c(sd.U, sd.U)` and `sd.U` is chosen
  as it is given in the present cell of the simulation grid.

The control parameter `crtl` is set to

`mob_control(objfun = function(object){-as.vector(logLik(object))})`.

This means that the control parameters of the MOB algorithm are set to the default
values, besides the `objfun` is set to the negative log-likelihood (cf. Section 3.2).
Via the `predict()` function the linear predictors for `train.data` and `test.data`
are computed, where via the argument `newdata` the test data is passed to the
`predict()` function. These vectors of the linear predictors as well as the censored
failure times for the training and test data, respectively, are passed to the `predErr()`
function. In addition, an user-specified time vector, which is here defined as a
sequence from 0 to the maximum of the failure time by 0.5, has to be specified. By

setting the type equal to "robust" the function predErr() returns the value of the estimated integrated prediction error ierror suggested by Schmid et al. (2011). The prediction error is only computed, if the true underlying tree structure is detected and the optimization did not fail. Because it makes only sense to compare the MOB with the global model consisting of the main effect and interaction effect, if the structural change in the MOB was truly estimated. Otherwise the prediction error of the MOB and the global model are set to NA. Again a variable count.NA is introduced, which counts the number of not detected true tree structures or failed optimizations.

The whole procedure is repeated 500 times, where in every repetition a new data set is simulated and is partitioned randomly in a training and test data set, so that in every run a new training and test data set is generated. Again the sample sizes 100, 500 and 1000 as well as the four different values of the error standard deviation sd.U are considered. The median and the 2.5% and 97.5% quantiles, which determine an approximate 95% confidence interval for the prediction error, are computed for the MOB and global model of each approach, respectively, whereby the $\lceil mc \cdot \alpha \rceil$ and $\lceil mc \cdot (1 - \alpha) \rceil$ value of the ordered sample provide the 2.5% and 97.5% quantiles with $\alpha = 0.025$ and mc = monte.carlo - count.NA. In addition boxplots are generated.

Results

The results for beta.1.true = 0.6, beta.2.true = -0.2 , tau.1.true = 0.5, tau.2.true = -0.4, prob.cens = 0% and $V_i \sim N(0, 1)$ are located in Appendix C.5.1. The boxplots of the prediction error for sample size 100, 500 and 1000 are shown in Figure C.55, C.56, C.57, C.58, C.59 and C.60 divided by the results for the global model and the MOB. The results for sd.U = 0 and sd.U = 0.1 are almost the same and in all cases the median of the prediction error of the MOB lies under the one of the global model. The different approaches perform in the same way. For sd.U = 0.4 and sd.U = 0.8 the MOB still shows in median lower values of the prediction error compared to the global models. For samples size 100 the prediction error of the corrected estimation is in median comparable to the benchmark estimation for the MOB and global model, respectively. For sample size 500 and 1000 the median prediction error lies over the benchmark estimation, for sd.U = 0.8 the difference is larger than for sd.U = 0.4. The naive estimator and the regression calibration show lower median prediction errors compared to the benchmark and corrected estimation for the MOB and global model, respectively. The interquartile range is smaller, but many extreme values are generated. For all sample sizes the naive estimator and the regression calibration result in the same boxplot, respectively.

The value of the median prediction error, named here as `ierror`, and the approximate 95% confidence interval `CI` for the global model and MOB are shown in Table C.43, C.44 and C.45 for sample size 100, 500 and 1000. In addition, the number of NAs (`#NA`) is printed. Here, no distinctions are made between not detected tree structures and failed optimizations. Having a look at the summary tables it can also be seen that the naive estimation and regression calibration result in exact the same results. This can be traced back to the definition of the regression calibration estimator. The linear predictors are integrated in the calculation of the prediction error and are in the case of the regression calibration given by

$$\hat{\beta}_0 + \hat{\beta}_{reg.calib} \cdot W_{reg.calib_i}, \tag{4.10}$$

which is equal to

$$\hat{\beta}_0 + \Sigma_V^{-1} \cdot (\Sigma_V + \Sigma_U) \cdot \hat{\beta}_{naive} \cdot [\mu_V + \Sigma_V \cdot (\Sigma_V + \Sigma_U)^{-1} \cdot (W_i - \mu_V)], \tag{4.11}$$

with $\hat{\beta}_{reg.calib} = \Sigma_V^{-1} \cdot (\Sigma_V + \Sigma_U) \cdot \hat{\beta}_{naive}$ and $W_{reg.calib_i} = \mu_V + \Sigma_V \cdot (\Sigma_V + \Sigma_U)^{-1} \cdot (W_i - \mu_V)$ (see Section 2.1.2). In the data generating process V is assumed to be normally distributed with mean zero and standard deviation of 1, thus $\mu_V = 0$ and $\Sigma_V = 1$. Substituting this in Equation (4.11) leads to

$$\hat{\beta}_0 + \hat{\beta}_{naive} \cdot W_i. \tag{4.12}$$

However, considering the results of the parameter estimation in the second part of the simulations study, the estimation of the naive estimator was biased and the corrected estimation shows comparable results to the benchmark estimation (see Section 4.2.1). Therefore, one would expect that the naive estimation results in worse prediction compared to the benchmark and corrected estimation. Here, it is the other way round. One explanation could be that due to the sampling of training and test data sets the observations in the trainings data set, which is used to estimate the prediction rule, do not follow the same distribution, which underlies in the whole simulated data set. At the consideration of a few single model outputs of the different approaches, it was observed that in some cases the benchmark and corrected estimation overestimate the true effect. The naive estimation is attenuated and is therefore closer to the true value of the parameter leading to a better prediction.

Considering the confidence intervals, it can be seen that the bounds for the corrected estimation are comparable to those of the benchmark estimation. Only for sd.U = 0.8 the range is shifted a little upwards. The naive approach and regression calibration result in the same confidence intervals, for the reason as described above, and result in comparable estimations to the benchmark and corrected estimation for sd.U = 0 and sd.U = 0.1. For sd.U = 0.4 and sd.U = 0.8 the bounds are smaller, at least for sample size 500 and 1000. However, the confidence intervals overlap, so that no significant difference in prediction accuracy can be shown for the different approaches.

The number of NAs (#NA) is rather high for sample size 100. Here, the problem is that due to estimating to MOB on the basis of only the training data set, thereby the sample size is reduced to 50, this means that 25 observations remain for each node. Therefore, the results of sample size 100 should be interpreted with caution. For increasing sample size this problem is overcome.

The results for 65% censoring are similar to those of 0%. For sample size 100 the number of NAs is again rather high and for sd.U = 0.8 the estimation of the upper bound of the confidence interval is Inf for the benchmark, naive and regression calibration approach. The results for 35% censoring are the other way round, here the global model results in lower prediction errors in comparison to the MOB. Again, the naive estimation and the regression calibration show in median lower prediction errors than the benchmark and corrected estimation.

The results for beta.1.true = 0.3, beta.2.true = 0.3 , tau.1.true = 0.5, tau.2.true = -0.4 (see the CD attatched to the appendix) show the same tendencies as the results described above, except for 35% censoring the MOB also results in lower prediction errors compared to the global model. Again, the results for sample size 100 need to be handled with caution. For 65% censoring the number of NAs is even over 420.

The results for beta.1.true = 0.6, beta.2.true = -0.2 , tau.1.true = 0.5, tau.2.true = 0.5 (see CD in the appendix) need to be taken with care, because for all sample sizes the number of NAs is rather high. For sample size 100 the number lies over 470, this means that the boxplots and the summary tables only base on 6% of the repetitions. For sample size 500 the number of NAs is 50%. For sample size 1000 between 70 and over 200 NAs are generated. Considering the results of sample size 1000 with the fewest number of NAs, it can be observed that the global model and the MOB results in comparable estimations. For sd.U = 0 and sd.U = 0.1 the results for the different approaches are similar. For higher error standard deviations the estimation of the naive and regression calibration results in lower prediction error compared to the benchmark estimation and corrected estimation. The corrected estimation results in most of the cases in a higher median of the estimated prediction errors, in some cases it lies below the benchmark estimation and in other cases the corrected estimation and benchmark estimation are comparable.

Conclusion

The results are quite heterogeneous. For some constellations the MOB results in a better prediction than the global model, for some the performance is comparable and for other constellations the MOB performs worse than the global model. All in all, the naive estimation shows a lower prediction error than the benchmark and corrected estimation. The regression calibration results in the exact same results as the naive estimation, which is due to the construction of regression calibration. The corrected estimation shows for some constellations comparable results to the benchmark estimation. In some situations it shows a higher prediction error compared to the benchmark approach.

Here, it would be interesting to compare the prediction error estimated by the robust Schemper-Henderson estimator to other suggested approaches, which estimates the prediction accuracy for survival data (see in the documentation of the package survAUC for other approaches and the corresponding references). In addition, larger sample sizes could be tested to overcome the problem of the high number of not detected true tree structures. The average and standard deviations of the resulting parameter estimation for the different approaches should be considered as well, to assess if by sampling the data set into training and test sets, the estimation differs from the resulting parameter estimation in the first and second part of the simulation study.

4.4. Conclusion of the Simulation Study

The integration of the corrected log-likelihood into the MOB algorithm works out well. The corrected parameter estimation in the terminal nodes are in mean close to the true parameter values. The test of parameter instability including the corrected score functions detect the underlying tree structure (in the case of a single partition).

For a low measurement error (sd.U = 0.1) the performance of the four approaches is quite similar and is comparable to the results with no measurement error (sd.U = 0). For no measurement error all approaches result in exact the same estimations, which is a verification for all approaches. Considering the resulting parameter estimation of the different approaches, which was examined in the first part of the simulation study. For higher measurement error (sd.U = 0.4 and sd.U = 0.8) the corrected estimation of β_V is comparable to the regression calibration. Compared to the benchmark estimation both approaches show a higher variability. The naive estimation is shifted, whereby the attenuation is larger for higher error variance. The estimation of the log-transformed scale parameter τ of the Weibull model differs for an increasing and decreasing hazard rate. In the case of an increasing hazard rate (negative τ) the corrected estimation is in mean equal to the benchmark estimation, but shows a higher variance. The naive estimation and regression calibration are shifted. In the case of a decreasing hazard rate (positive τ) the corrected and regression calibration result in comparable estimations and are in mean close to the benchmark estimation. Here, only the naive estimation is shifted. This suggests that in the case of an increasing hazard rate the corrected estimation is the most reliable estimation. Here, the estimation is in mean better than for the regression calibration and the naive estimation, but a higher variance has to be accepted (variance-bias-trade-off). For a decreasing hazard rate the results of the corrected estimation and regression calibration show comparable results. The inclusion of an error-free covariable works out well.

The new implemented sandwich estimator, which estimates the variance of the corrected estimation, turns out to be approximately equal to the sample variance. The optimization of the corrected log-likelihood via the optim() function failed for some constellations, mainly for sd.U = 0.8 and sample size 100.

Considering the inclusion of the corrected score functions in the MOB algorithm, to assess parameter instability, the detection rate for a true underlying tree was examined in the second part of the simulation study. It turns out that the detection rate of a single structural change for a binary partitioning variable is comparable for all approaches. This privides evidence that the corrected MOB algorithm results in similar detection rates compared to the naive estimation and regression calibration as well as the benchmark estimation. Only in the case of sd.U = 0.8 problems with the optimization occur for the corrected approach and thus the detection rate is lower than for the other approaches. All in all, it can be seen that the larger the sample size, the higher is the detection rate. Moreover, the results suggest that a structural change is easier to detect for a difference in τ than for a difference in β. The resulting parameter estimation in the terminal nodes is similar to the separate consideration of the fit function in the first part of the simulation study.

For the consideration of more than one structural change the detection rate turns out to be rather low, where the different approaches perform in a comparable way. Therefore, this problem cannot be traced back to the corrected MOB algorithm. It seems to be a problem to detect structures which are close to the XOR problem. This provides evidence that better results are obtained for simple partitions, and for larger sample sizes. In general, small sample sizes turn out to be a problem in fitting the MOB algorithm. Structural changes are not detected, because the number of observations is too small to build up the terminal nodes.

In the third part of the simulation study the prediction accuracy of the MOB is compared to a global model. The results are quite heterogeneous. For some constellations the MOB performs better than the global model, in other constellations, it is the other way round. Again, for a low measurement error ($\mathtt{sd.U} = 0.1$) the four approaches perform in a similar way within the MOB and global model, respectively. The results are comparable to the results with no measurement error. For increasing error variance it turns out that the naive estimation shows the lowest prediction error compared to the corrected and benchmark estimation, which was not expected by observing a biased estimation of the naive estimation in the first and second part of the simulation study. The regression calibration results in exact the same prediction errors as the naive estimation, which is due to the construction of the regression calibration approach. The corrected estimator results in higher prediction errors compared to the naive and regression calibration approach. For some constellations the prediction error is higher than for the benchmark estimation, for others the performance is comparable to the benchmark estimation. Because of the quite heterogeneous results, this part of the simulation study should be validated for example via other approaches to estimate the prediction error for survival data and with larger sample sizes.

5. Conclusion

Within the framework of this thesis the MOB algorithm for the Weibull model is extended, such that a corrected parameter estimation for the Weibull model within the MOB algorithm can be considered. In Chapter 2 the incorporation of the adjustment for measurement error is derived theoretically. On the basis of this it is integrated into the `mob()` function, described in detail in Chapter 3. The correction for measurement error is incorporated in the four steps of the MOB algorithm: In the first step of the parameter estimation the derived corrected log-likelihood of the Weibull model is implemented in a new fit function called `SurvRegcorr@fit()`, which optimizes the corrected log-likelihood via the `optim()` function. A new object `SurvRegcorr` of class `StatModel` is implemented, where the new implemented `SurvRegcorr@fit()` function is attached. The whole procedure is implemented in such a way that the returned object is comparable to the one of the function `survreg()`, which fits an uncorrected Weibull model, so that the model summaries can be generated to consider the resulting parameter estimates as well as their inference. In the second step the corrected score function of the Weibull is embedded into the empirical fluctuation process, which is used to compute the test statistic to asses the parameter instability. The optimal split point is found by maximizing the partitioned corrected log-likelihood of the Weibull model in the third step. The last step re-fits the model again by the implemented fit function `SurvRegcorr@fit()`.

The existing `mob()` function can be used in a familiar way. To fit a corrected Weibull model the `model` argument has to be set to `SurvRegcorr`. Furthermore, the variables measured with error and the error standard deviations have to be specified in `error.var` and `sd.U`, respectively.

Practical problems arise by fitting the corrected Weibull model via the `mob()` function. By optimizing the corrected log-likelihood via the `optim()` function the running time is extended seriously. To find the optimal split point the fitted model is `reweight()`ed for every possible split point. This means that the `optim()` function is called every time, when `reweight()` is conducted. Considering a categorical partitioning variable the problem is less serious, because the possible split points are only a few and in the case of a binary splitting variable the split point is trivial. Thus, the running time of the `mob()` function depends on the model complexity as well as how many nodes are detected and which types of partitioning variables are selected for splitting.

In Chapter 4, a simulation study is conducted to analyse the performance of the new implemented fit function, which is compared to the benchmark estimation, the naive estimation and to the regression calibration. The performance is evaluated in three parts. At first, the performance of the new implemented `fit` function `SurvRegcorr@fit()` is analysed separately. Secondly, the behaviour of `SurvRegcorr@fit()` within the MOB algorithm as well as the detection rate for the true underlying tree structure is examined. Thirdly, the prediction accuracy of a global model and a MOB are compared.

The integration of the corrected log-likelihood into the MOB algorithm works out well. The corrected parameter estimation in the terminal nodes is in mean close to the true parameter values. In addition, the inclusion of an error-free covariable works out well. The test of parameter instability including the corrected score functions detects the underlying tree structure (in the case of a single partition).

For a low measurement error the performance of the naive estimation, corrected estimation and regression calibration is quite similar and is comparable to the results with no measurement error. This suggests that the consideration of the corrected parameter estimation is not necessary in this case. For higher measurement error the corrected approach still provides an unbiased estimation in contrast to the naive estimation. Considering only the parameter estimation of β the regression calibration performs in a comparable way to the corrected estimation. For the estimation of τ the regression calibration differs from the corrected estimation. In the case of an increasing hazard rate (negative τ) the regression calibration leads to biased estimation. In the case of a decreasing hazard rate (positive τ) the regression calibration results in comparable estimation. This suggests that in the case of an increasing hazard rate the corrected estimation is the most reliable estimation, it is in mean better than for the regression calibration and the naive estimation, but a higher variance has to be accepted (variance-bias-trade-off). For a decreasing hazard rate the results of the corrected estimation and regression calibration show comparable results.

The separate consideration of the estimation accuracy for the fit function in the first part of the simulation study is comparable to the one in the terminal nodes of the resulting tree in the second part.

The deficit of the corrected approach is that the optimization via the `optim()` function failed for some constellations, mainly for a higher error variance and sample size 100.

Analysing more than one structural change, results in unsatisfactory findings. Only a few true underlying tree structures are detected by the MOB algorithm in the repeated runs, but the different approaches perform in a comparable way, so that this problem cannot be traced back to the new implemented corrected MOB algorithm. Comparing the prediction error between a MOB and a global model results in heterogeneous performance. Here, further analyses have to be conducted.

To validate the hypotheses of the simulation study further investigations should be carried out.

Outlook

In Chapter 2, the incorporation of the corrected estimation for the Cox model into the MOB algorithm is only considered theoretically. The implementation would be conducted analogue to the corrected Weibull model (cf. Section 3.2). At first, it is reasonable to integrate the uncorrected Cox model into the `mob()` function, because a model-based parameter estimation is only possible for the Weibull model so far. This would also be useful to compare the corrected approach to the uncorrected one in a simulation study. For that a new object say `CoxPH` of class `StatModel` is generated according to `survReg`. The `fit` function has to be modified in that way that the model is fitted via the `coxph()` function from the package `survival`. This is the usual function to fit a Cox model in R. By default the Efron approximation is used to adjust for ties. To make the results comparable to the corrected approach the Breslow method should be used. Therefore, the argument `method` is set to `"breslow"`. The modified `fit` function should return an object of class `CoxPH` and `coxph`. This is important, so that further functions can be implemented for the new object and functions, which are already available for an object of class `coxph`, can be inherited to an object of class `CoxPH`. For the test of parameter instability a function `estfun()` is required to extract the values of the score function of the Cox model evaluated at the parameter estimators. In the package `sandwich` (Zeileis, 2006) `estfun.coxph()` is already available and can be used here. In addition, a function `weights.CoxPH()` is needed to extract the

weights of the fitted model object. This function can be implemented analogue
to `weights.survReg()`. To find the optimal split point, two functions have to be
implemented. A function `logLik.CoxPH()` extracts the value of the log-likelihood
of the Cox model, and a function `reweight.CoxPH()` re-fits the fitted model. Again,
this can be conducted analogue to `logLik.survReg()` and `reweight.survReg()`.
In addition, the `print()` function has to be adopted to the new object specified by
`print.CoxPH()`.

To fit a MOB tree based on a Cox model with adjustment for measurement error,
a new object `CoxPHcorr` of class `StatModel` is implemented. A new `fit` function,
which is attached to the new object `CoxPHcorr` via the `@`-operator, should include
the optimization of the corrected log-likelihood from the Cox model (see Equation
(2.24)) via the `optim()` function. Assuming normal homoscedastic errors, $M_U(\beta_X)$
is chosen as in Equation (2.27). The baseline hazard rate has to be estimated
in addition to β_X, instead of the scale parameter of the Weibull model. For the
inference on the estimated parameters the sandwich estimator of the variance has to
be computed (see Equation (2.28)). Therefore, the corrected score functions of β_X
from Equation (2.25) and of h_j (see Appendix B.2) have to be implemented. The
estimated variance can be used to compute the Wald test from Equation (2.33) and
the likelihood ratio test from Equation (2.34) for the model summary. The returned
object of `CoxPHcorr@fit()` is allocated to two classes `CoxPHcorr` and `coxph`. For
the parameter instability test an `estfun.CoxPHcorr()` function, which returns a
matrix with the values of the corrected score functions for β_X and for the baseline
hazard rate as defined in Equation (2.25) and in Appendix B.2, respectively, as
well as a `weights.CoxPHcorr()` function is required. The `weights()` function
can be implemented analogue to `weights.survReg()`. The optimal split point is
determined via the maximal partitioned corrected log-likelihood of the Cox model.
To extract the value of the corrected log-likelihood of the Cox model, a function
`logLik.CoxPHcorr()` has to be implemented. To re-fit the Cox model via the
corrected log-likelihood, a function `reweight.CoxPHcorr()` is needed. It can be
implemented analogue to `reweight.survReg()`. Finally, the `print()` function has
to be modified for the new object `CoxPHcorr`.

The `mob()` function can again be used in a familiar way. To fit a model-based
Cox model to survival data, the `model` argument has to be set to `CoxPH`. The
usual functions such as `summary()`, `print()` and `plot()` can be applied to the
returned object of class `mob`. If one fits a model-based Cox model with adjustment
for measurement error, the `model` argument in the `mob()` function has to be set to

CoxPHcorr. In addition, the variables measured with error and the error standard deviations have to be specified in error.var and sd.U, respectively.

The MOB algorithm requires an unbiased estimating function. Therefore, a correction for measurement error could be included in the MOB algorithm for almost every generalized linear model, if a corrected score function or a corrected log-likelihood can be derived, which fulfils the condition (2.12) or (2.13) of being an unbiased estimation equation (see for example Nakamura (1990), who started with the development of corrected score functions in generalized linear models).

A. R-Code

A.1. *SurvRegcorr.r*

The file *SurvRegcorr.r* contains the new implemented function `SurvRegcorr@fit()`.
The function provides a corrected model fit for the Weibull model. This includes an
optimization of the corrected log-likelihood under the assumption of homoscedastic
normal measurement errors from Equation (2.58) via the `optim()` function. The
following arguments are passed to the function: `object` is an object of class
`ModelEnvFormula` including the model `formula` and the `data`. `weights` is an
optional vector of weights to be used in the fitting process. In `error.var` and `sd.U`
the covariables measured with error and the standard deviation of the errors are
specified, respectively.

```r
1  SurvRegcorr@fit <- function(object, weights = NULL, error.var = error.var,
2                              sd.U = sd.U, ...)
3  {
4
5    if(missing(error.var)){
6      stop("error.var is missing!")
7    }else{
8      if(!is.character(error.var)){
9      stop("error.var must be a string!")
10     }
11   }
12
13   if(missing(sd.U)){
14     stop("sd.U is missing!")
15   }
16
17   if(length(sd.U) != length(error.var)){
18     stop("length(sd.U) != length(error.var)")
19   }
20
21   if(length(intersect(names(object@get("input")), error.var)) == 0){
```

```
22      stop("error.var does not match one of the passed covariable(s)!")
23    }
24
25    ### data preparation
26
27    Y <- object@get("response")
28    names(Y) <- "y"
29
30    W <- object@get("input")[, error.var]
31    W <- as.data.frame(W)
32    names(W) <- error.var
33
34    if(length(error.var) == dim(object@get("input"))[2]){
35      Z <- NULL
36      mydata <- cbind (Y,W)
37    }else{
38      Z <- object@get("input")[,-c(match(error.var,
39       names(object@get("input"))))]
40      if(dim(object@get("input"))[2] - length(error.var) == 1){
41          Z <- as.data.frame(Z)
42          names(Z) <- names(object@get("input"))[-c(match(error.var,
43           names(object@get("input"))))]}
44      mydata <- cbind (Y,W,Z)
45    }
46
47    if (!is.null(weights)){
48      mydata <- mydata[weights > 0, ]
49      weights <- weights[weights > 0]
50    }
51
52    time <- mydata$y[,1]
53    event <- mydata$y[,2]   # 0 = alive, 1 = dead
54
55    k <- sum(event)          # number of events
56    n <- length(event)       # number of observations
57
58    # design matrix
59    A <- cbind(Intercept = rep(1,dim(mydata)[1]),mydata[,-1])
60    A <- as.data.frame(A)
61    if(is.null(dim(mydata[,-1]))){
62      names(A)[2] <- error.var
63    }
64
```

```
65    ### minus corrected log-likelihood
66
67    minus.log.lik.weibull <- function(model.par)
68    {
69
70      betaX <- model.par[1:dim(A)[2]]
71      tau <- model.par[dim(A)[2]+1]
72
73      rval <- sum((((log(time) - t(betaX %*% t(A)))/exp(tau)) - tau -
74              log(time))[event == 1]) - sum(exp((log(time)/exp(tau)) -
75              apply((((betaX * t(A))/exp(tau)) + (M.U(family = "normal",
76              sd.U = sd.U, beta = betaX)/exp(tau)^2)), 2, sum)))
77
78      return(-rval)
79
80    }
81
82    ### corrected score functions
83
84    score.corr.beta <- function(par)
85    {
86
87      betaX <- par[1:dim(A)[2]]
88      tau <- par[dim(A)[2]+1]
89
90      A.neu <- A
91      A.neu[event != 1,] <- 0
92      rval <- (1/exp(tau)) * (exp((log(time)/exp(tau)) - apply(((((betaX *
93              t(A))/exp(tau)) + (M.U(family = "normal", sd.U = sd.U,
94              beta = betaX)/exp(tau)^2)), 2, sum)) * t(t(A) +
95              (d.log.M.U(family = "normal", sd.U = sd.U,
96              beta = betaX)/exp(tau))) - A.neu)
97      return(rval)
98
99    }
100
101
102    score.corr.log.scale <- function(par)
103    {
104
105      betaX <- par[1:dim(A)[2]]
106      tau <- par[dim(A)[2]+1]
107
```

```
108    c1 <- 1 + ((log(time) - t(betaX %*% t(A)))/exp(tau))
109    c1[event != 1] <- 0
110
111    rval <- -c1 + ((exp((log(time)/exp(tau)) - apply(((((betaX *
112            t(A))/exp(tau)) + (M.U(family = "normal", sd.U = sd.U, beta =
113            betaX)/exp(tau)^2)), 2, sum))) * ((log(time)/exp(tau)) -
114            apply(((((betaX * t(A))/exp(tau)) + (2* M.U(family = "normal",
115            sd.U = sd.U, beta = betaX)/exp(tau)^2)), 2, sum)))
116
117    rval <- as.data.frame(rval)
118    names(rval) <- "Log(scale)"
119
120    return(rval)
121
122  }
123
124  ### moment generating function
125
126  M.U <- function(family = "normal", sd.U, beta)
127  {
128
129    if(family == "normal"){
130      rval <- rep(0, length(beta))
131      rval[2:(1+length(error.var))] <- (sd.U^2 *
132                       beta[2:(1+length(error.var))]^2)/2
133    }
134
135    return(rval)
136
137  }
138
139  d.log.M.U <- function(family = "normal", sd.U, beta)
140  {
141
142    if(family == "normal"){
143      rval <- rep(0, length(beta))
144      rval[2:(1+length(error.var))] <- sd.U^2 *
145          beta[2:(1+length(error.var))]
146    }
147
148    return(rval)
149  }
150
```

```
151    ### start values
152
153    survreg.naive <- survreg(y ~ ., data = mydata, dist = "weibull",
154                             weights = weights)
155
156    # null model
157    survreg.null <- survreg(y ~ 1, data = mydata, dist = "weibull",
158                            weights = weights)
159
160    # start value for beta
161    betaX.start <- as.numeric(survreg.naive$coef)
162
163    # start value for tau (log(scale))
164    tau.start <- log(as.numeric(survreg.naive$scale))
165
166    model.par.naive <- c(betaX.start, tau.start)
167
168    ### optimization
169
170    rval <- optim(model.par.naive, minus.log.lik.weibull,
171              method = "Nelder-Mead" , hessian = TRUE)
172
173    ### preparation for output
174
175    # coefficients
176    coef.model <- rval$par[1:(length(rval$par)-1)]
177    names(coef.model) <- c(names(A))
178    coef0 <- c(as.numeric(survreg.null$coef), log(survreg.null$scale))
179    names(coef0) <- c("Intercept", "Log(scale)")
180
181    # variance (robust sandwich estimator)
182    hess <- rval$hessian
183    dimnames(hess) <- list(c(names(A),"Log(scale)"),
184        c(names(A),"Log(scale)"))
185    hessinv <- solve(hess)
186    score <- cbind(score.corr.beta(rval$par),
187     score.corr.log.scale(rval$par))
188    score <- as.matrix(score)
189    C <- crossprod(score)   # = C <- t(score) %*% score
190    var <- hessinv %*% C %*% hessinv
191    # linear predictors: x'beta
192    lin.pred <- as.vector(as.matrix(A) %*% coef.model)
193    dimnames(lin.pred) <- NULL
```

```
194
195    # call
196    mycall <- quote(optim(model.par.naive,minus.log.lik.weibull,
197                    method = "Nelder-Mead",hessian=TRUE))
198
199    # terms
200    Terms <- survreg.naive$terms
201
202    # y
203    transy <- cbind(log(mydata$y[,1]),mydata$y[,2])
204    dimnames(transy) <- list(dimnames(mydata)[[1]], NULL)
205
206    # output
207    z <- list(coefficients = coef.model, icoef = coef0, var = var,
208            loglik = c(survreg.null$loglik[1], -rval$value),
209            iter = as.integer(rval$counts[1]), linear.predictors
210            = lin.pred, df = as.integer(length(coef.model)+ 1),
211            scale = exp(rval$par[length(rval$par)]), idf = length(coef0),
212            df.residual = as.integer(n - (length(coef.model) + 1)),
213            terms =  Terms, means = apply(A,2,mean), call = mycall,
214            dist = "weibull", y = transy,
215            error.var = error.var, sd.U = sd.U, emp.estfun.corr =
216            as.matrix(cbind(score.corr.beta(rval$par),
217            score.corr.log.scale(rval$par)))
218            )
219
220    z$ModelEnv <- object
221    z$addargs <- list(...)
222    z$weights <- weights
223    class(z) <- c("SurvRegcorr", "survreg")
224    return(z)
225
226  }
```

B. Proofs and Derivations

B.1. Cox Model - Corrected Log-Likelihood

The corrected log-likelihood from Equation (2.24) has to fulfil the condition of being an unbiased estimation equation. Under the assumption of an additive measurement error model it has to be shown that $\mathbb{E}(l^A_{corr}(\pi, A, \beta_X, h_j)|V, F, \tilde{Y}) = l^X_{Br}(\pi, X, \beta_X, h_j)$ (see Equation 2.13).

$$
\mathbb{E}(l^A_{corr}(\pi, A, \beta_X, h_j)|V, F, \tilde{Y})
$$

$$
= \mathbb{E}\left(\sum_{j=1}^{k} \left[d_j ln(h_j) + \sum_{i \in D(\pi_j)} \beta'_X A_i - h_j(\pi_j - \pi_{j-1}) \cdot \right.\right.
$$

$$
\left.\left. \sum_{i \in R(\pi_j)} \frac{exp(\beta'_X A_i)}{M_{U_i}(\beta_X)} \right] \middle| V, F, \tilde{Y} \right)
$$

$$
= \mathbb{E}\left(\sum_{j=1}^{k} \left[d_j ln(h_j) + \sum_{i \in D(\pi_j)} (\beta'_V W_i + \beta'_F F_i) - h_j(\pi_j - \pi_{j-1}) \cdot \right.\right.
$$

$$
\left.\left. \sum_{i \in R(\pi_j)} \frac{exp(\beta'_V W_i + \beta'_F F_i)}{M_{U_i}(\beta_X)} \right] \middle| V, F, \tilde{Y} \right)
$$

$$
= \mathbb{E}\left(\sum_{j=1}^{k} \left[d_j ln(h_j) + \sum_{i \in D(\pi_j)} (\beta'_V (V_i + U_i) + \beta'_F F_i) - h_j(\pi_j - \pi_{j-1}) \cdot \right.\right.
$$

$$
\left.\left. \sum_{i \in R(\pi_j)} \frac{exp(\beta'_V (V_i + U_i) + \beta'_F F_i)}{M_{U_i}(\beta_X)} \right] \middle| V, F, \tilde{Y} \right)
$$

$$
\overset{U_i \perp (V_i, F_i)}{=} \mathbb{E}\left(\sum_{j=1}^{k} \left[d_j ln(h_j) + \sum_{i \in D(\pi_j)} (\beta'_V V_i + \beta'_V U_i + \beta'_F F_i) - h_j(\pi_j - \pi_{j-1}) \cdot \right.\right.
$$

$$
\left.\left. \sum_{i \in R(\pi_j)} \frac{exp(\beta'_V V_i + \beta'_V U_i + \beta'_F F_i)}{M_{U_i}(\beta_V) \cdot M_{U_i}(\beta_F)} \right] \middle| V, F, \tilde{Y} \right)
$$

$$= \sum_{j=1}^{k} \left[d_j ln(h_j) + \sum_{i \in D(\pi_j)} \beta'_V V_i + \sum_{i \in D(\pi_j)} \mathbb{E}(\beta'_V U_i | V, F, \tilde{Y}) + \sum_{i \in D(\pi_j)} \beta'_F F_i - \right.$$

$$\left. h_j(\pi_j - \pi_{j-1}) \cdot \sum_{i \in R(\pi_j)} \frac{exp(\beta'_V V_i)}{M_{U_i}(\beta_V)} \cdot \mathbb{E}(exp(\beta'_V U_i) | V, F, \tilde{Y}) \cdot \frac{exp(\beta'_F F_i)}{M_{U_i}(\beta_F)} \right]$$

$$\overset{(B.1),(B.2)}{=} \sum_{j=1}^{k} \left[d_j ln(h_j) + \sum_{i \in D(\pi_j)} \beta'_V V_i + \sum_{i \in D(\pi_j)} \beta'_F F_i - h_j(\pi_j - \pi_{j-1}) \cdot \right.$$

$$\left. \sum_{i \in R(\pi_j)} \frac{exp(\beta'_V V_i)}{M_{U_i}(\beta_V)} \cdot M_{U_i}(\beta_V) \cdot \frac{exp(\beta'_F F_i)}{M_{U_i}(\beta_F)} \right]$$

$$\overset{(B.3)}{=} \sum_{j=1}^{k} \left[d_j ln(h_j) + \sum_{i \in D(\pi_j)} (\beta'_V V_i + \beta'_F F_i) - h_j(\pi_j - \pi_{j-1}) \cdot \right.$$

$$\left. \sum_{i \in R(\pi_j)} exp(\beta'_V V_i + \beta'_F F_i) \right]$$

$$= \sum_{j=1}^{k} \left[d_j ln(h_j) + \sum_{i \in D(\pi_j)} \beta'_X X_i - h_j(\pi_j - \pi_{j-1}) \cdot \sum_{i \in R(\pi_j)} exp(\beta'_X X_i) \right]$$

$$= l_{Br}^{X}(\pi, X, \beta_X, h_j)$$

Given that U_i is independent of V_i, F_i, T_i and δ_i, $i = 1, \ldots n$, the following is used in the proof

$$\mathbb{E}(\beta'_V U_i | V, F, \tilde{Y}) = \mathbb{E}(\beta'_V U_i) = 0 \tag{B.1}$$

$$\mathbb{E}(exp(\beta'_V U_i) | V, F, \tilde{Y}) = \mathbb{E}(exp(\beta'_V U_i)) = M_{U_i}(\beta_V). \tag{B.2}$$

Because F_i denotes error free covariable(s), the corresponding moment generating function is set to 1:

$$M_{U_i}(\beta_F) = 1. \tag{B.3}$$

By the law of iterated expectation it follows that $\mathbb{E}(l_{corr}^{A}(\pi, A, \beta_X, h_j) | V, F, \tilde{Y}) = 0$ (cf. Equation (2.15)).

B.2. Cox Model - Corrected Score Functions

In Appendix B.1 it was shown that the corrected log-likelihood from Equation (2.24) fulfils the condition of being an unbiased estimation equation. Condition (2.12) implies that the differentiation with respect to the parameters provides the according corrected score function(s). Here, the corrected score functions are the derivatives of $l_{corr}^A(\pi, A, \beta_X, h_j)$ with respect to $h_1, \ldots, h_k$ and β_X. For h_j the corrected score function is derived as follows

$$\frac{\partial l_{corr}^A(\pi, A, \beta_X)}{\partial h_j} = \left[\frac{d_j}{h_j} - (\pi_j - \pi_{j-1}) \sum_{i \in R(\pi_j)} \frac{exp(\beta_X' A_i)}{M_{U_i}(\beta_X)} \right], \quad j = 1, \ldots, k,$$

and the corresponding root is

$$\hat{h}_j = \frac{d_j}{(\pi_j - \pi_{j-1}) \sum_{i \in R(\pi_j)} exp(\hat{\beta}_X' A_i)/M_{U_i}(\hat{\beta}_X)} . \tag{B.4}$$

Then, in dependence on β

$$\hat{H}_0(t) = \int_0^t \sum_{j=1}^k \hat{h}_j \cdot 1_{\pi_{j-1} < t \le \pi_j} du = \sum_{j: \pi_j \le t} \frac{d_j}{\sum_{i \in R(\pi_j)} exp(\hat{\beta}_X' A_i)/M_{U_i}(\hat{\beta}_X)} .$$

For β_X one obtains

$$\frac{\partial l_{corr}^A(\pi, A, \beta_X)}{\partial \beta_X} = \sum_{j=1}^k \left(\sum_{i \in D(\pi_j)} A_i - h_j(\pi_j - \pi_{j-1}) \right) \cdot$$
$$\left(\sum_{i \in R(\pi_j)} \frac{A_i \cdot exp(\beta_X' A_i) \cdot M_{U_i}(\beta_X) - \frac{\partial}{\partial \beta_X} M_{U_i}(\beta_X) \cdot exp(\beta_X' A_i)}{(M_{U_i}(\beta_X))^2} \right)$$

$$\stackrel{(B.4)}{=} \sum_{j=1}^k \left(\sum_{i \in D(\pi_j)} A_i - \frac{d_j}{\sum_{i \in R(\pi_j)} exp(\beta_X' A_i)/M_{U_i}(\beta_X)} \right) \cdot$$
$$\left(\sum_{i \in R(\pi_j)} exp(\beta_X' A_i)/M_{U_i}(\beta_X) \cdot \left(A_i - \frac{\partial}{\partial \beta_X} M_{U_i}(\beta_X)/M_{U_i}(\beta_X) \right) \right)$$

and with

$$\frac{\frac{\partial}{\partial \beta_X} M_{U_i}(\beta_X)}{M_{U_i}(\beta_X)} = \frac{\partial}{\partial \beta_X} ln M_{U_i}(\beta_X)$$

leads to Equation (2.25).

B.3. Weibull Model - Log-Likelihood

The model equation and the log-likelihood for the Weibull model can be set up in two different ways. The first version is motivated by the semi-parametric Cox model (see Equation (2.42)). The second version is given Appendix B.3.1. However, it can be shown that both versions are equivalent (see Appendix B.3.2).

B.3.1. Version 2

The log-likelihood for the second version is given as follows (see Fahrmeir et al., 1996, Chapter 7).

$$l^X(\pi, X, \beta_X, \nu) = \sum_{i=1}^{n} \left[-\delta_i ln(\nu) + \delta_i log(h(y_i)) + log(S(y_i)) \right],$$

and with Equation (2.44) and (2.45) the log-likelihood can be transformed into

$$= \sum_{i=1}^{n} \left[-\delta_i ln(\nu) + \delta_i log \left(\frac{1}{\nu} exp \left(\frac{y_i - \theta_i}{\nu} \right) \right) + log \left(exp \left(-exp \left(\frac{y_i - \theta_i}{\nu} \right) \right) \right) \right]$$

$$= \sum_{i=1}^{n} \left[-\delta_i ln(\nu) + \delta_i(-log(\nu)) + \delta_i \left(\frac{y_i - \theta_i}{\nu} \right) - exp \left(\frac{y_i - \theta_i}{\nu} \right) \right]$$

$$= \sum_{i=1}^{n} \left[-2 \cdot \delta_i ln(\nu) + \delta_i \left(\frac{y_i - \theta_i}{\nu} \right) - exp \left(\frac{y_i - \theta_i}{\nu} \right) \right]$$

$$\propto \sum_{i=1}^{n} \left[\delta_i \left[\left(\frac{y_i - \theta_i}{\nu} \right) - ln(\nu) \right] - exp \left(\frac{y_i - \theta_i}{\nu} \right) \right]$$

$$\overset{\tau = ln(\nu)}{=} \sum_{i=1}^{n} \left[\delta_i \left[\left(\frac{y_i - \beta_X' X_i}{exp(\tau)} \right) - \tau \right] - exp \left(\frac{y_i - \beta_X' X_i}{exp(\tau)} \right) \right].$$

B.3.2. Version 2 = Version 1

It is shown that the second version (Equation (2.47)) and first version (Equation(2.42)) of the log-likelihood for the Weibull model are equivalent. Starting with Equation (2.47):

$$\sum_{i=1}^{n} \left[\delta_i \left[\left(\frac{y_i - \theta_i}{\nu} \right) - ln(\nu) \right] - exp \left(\frac{y_i - \theta_i}{\nu} \right) \right]$$

$$= \sum_{i=1}^{n} \left[\delta_i \left[\left(\frac{ln(t_i) - \beta_X' X_i}{\nu} \right) - ln(\nu) \right] - exp \left(\frac{ln(t_i) - \beta_X' X_i}{\nu} \right) \right]$$

$$= \sum_{i=1}^{n} \left[\delta_i \left[\frac{1}{\nu} ln(t_i) - \frac{\beta_X' X_i}{\nu} - ln(\nu) \right] - exp \left(\frac{1}{\nu} ln(t_i) - \frac{\beta_X' X_i}{\nu} \right) \right]$$

$$= \sum_{i=1}^{n} \left[\delta_i \left[ln(t_i)^{1/\nu} + \beta_X^{+'} X_i - ln(\nu) \right] - t_i^{1/\nu} exp(\beta_X^{+'} X_i) \right]$$

$$= \sum_{i=1}^{n} \left[\delta_i \left[ln \left(\frac{1}{\nu} \cdot t_i^{1/\nu} \right) + \beta_X^{+'} X_i \right] - t_i^{1/\nu} exp(\beta_X^{+'} X_i) \right]$$

with $\beta_X^+ = -\beta_X / \nu$. Add the term $-log(t_i)$, which does not depend on β or ν and can be left out, because of proportionality. This leads to the first version (Equation (2.42)):

$$= \sum_{i=1}^{n} \left[\delta_i \left[ln \left(\frac{1}{\nu} \cdot t_i^{1/\nu} \right) - log(t_i) + \beta_X^{+'} X_i \right] - t_i^{1/\nu} exp(\beta_X^{+'} X_i) \right]$$

$$= \sum_{i=1}^{n} \left[\delta_i \left[ln \left(\frac{1}{\nu} \cdot t_i^{1/\nu-1} \right) + \beta_X^{+'} X_i \right] - t_i^{1/\nu} exp(\beta_X^{+'} X_i) \right]$$

B.4. Weibull Model - Corrected Log-Likelihood

The corrected log-likelihood of the Weibull model is derived in Equation (2.49). The corrected log-likelihood has to fulfil the condition (2.13) of unbiased estimation. Under the assumption of an additive measurement error model it has to be shown that $\mathbb{E}(l_{corr}^A(t, A, \beta_X, \tau) | V, F, \tilde{Y}) = l^X(t, X, \beta_X, \tau)$.

$$\mathbb{E}(l_{corr}^A(t, A, \beta_X, \tau) | V, F, \tilde{Y})$$

$$= \mathbb{E} \left(\sum_{i=1}^{n} \left[\delta_i \left[\left(\frac{y_i - \beta_X' A_i}{exp(\tau)} \right) - \tau \right] - exp \left(\frac{y_i - \beta_X' A_i}{exp(\tau)} - ln(M_{U_i}(\beta_X^+)) \right) \right] \middle| V, F, \tilde{Y} \right)$$

$$= \mathbb{E} \left(\sum_{i=1}^{n} \left[\delta_i \left[\left(\frac{y_i - (\beta_0 + \beta_V' W_i + \beta_F' F_i)}{exp(\tau)} \right) - \tau \right] - \right. \right.$$
$$\left. \left. exp \left(\frac{y_i - (\beta_0 + \beta_V' W_i + \beta_F' F_i)}{exp(\tau)} - ln(M_{U_i}(\beta_X^+)) \right) \right] \middle| V, F, \tilde{Y} \right)$$

$$= \mathbb{E} \left(\sum_{i=1}^{n} \left[\delta_i \left[\left(\frac{y_i - \beta_0 - \beta_V'(V_i + U_i) - \beta_F' F_i}{exp(\tau)} \right) - \tau \right] - \right. \right.$$

$$exp\left(\frac{y_i - \beta_0 - \beta_V'(V_i + U_i) - \beta_F'F_i}{exp(\tau)} - ln(M_{U_i}(\beta_X^+))\right)\Bigg]\Bigg|\ V, F, \tilde{Y}\ \right)$$

$$= \mathbb{E}\left(\ \sum_{i=1}^{n}\left[\ \delta_i\left[\left(\frac{y_i - \beta_0 - \beta_V'V_i - \beta_V'U_i - \beta_F'F_i}{exp(\tau)}\right) - \tau\right] - \right.\right.$$

$$exp\left(\frac{y_i - \beta_0 - \beta_V'V_i - \beta_V'U_i - \beta_F'F_i}{exp(\tau)} - ln(M_{U_i}(\beta_X^+))\right)\Bigg]\Bigg|\ V, F, \tilde{Y}\ \right)$$

$$= \mathbb{E}\left(\ \sum_{i=1}^{n}\left[\ \delta_i\left[\left(\frac{y_i - \beta_0 - \beta_V'V_i - \beta_F'F_i}{exp(\tau)} - \frac{\beta_V'U_i}{exp(\tau)}\right) - \tau\right] - \right.\right.$$

$$exp\left(\frac{y_i - \beta_0 - \beta_V'V_i - \beta_F'F_i}{exp(\tau)} - \frac{\beta_V'U_i}{exp(\tau)} - ln(M_{U_i}(\beta_X^+))\right)\Bigg]\Bigg|\ V, F, \tilde{Y}\ \right)$$

$$\overset{B.7}{=} \mathbb{E}\left(\ \sum_{i=1}^{n}\left[\ \delta_i\left[\left(\frac{y_i - \beta_0 - \beta_V'V_i - \beta_F'F_i}{exp(\tau)} - \frac{\beta_V'U_i}{exp(\tau)}\right) - \tau\right] - \right.\right.$$

$$exp\left(\frac{y_i - \beta_0 - \beta_V'V_i - \beta_F'F_i}{exp(\tau)}\right) \cdot exp\left(-\frac{\beta_V'U_i}{exp(\tau)}\right) \cdot$$

$$exp\left(-ln(M_{U_i}(\beta_V^+))\right)\Bigg]\Bigg|\ V, F, \tilde{Y}\ \right)$$

$$= \sum_{i=1}^{n}\left[\ \delta_i\left[\left(\frac{y_i - \beta_0 - \beta_V'V_i - \beta_F'F_i}{exp(\tau)}\right) + \mathbb{E}\left(\left(-\frac{\beta_V'U_i}{exp(\tau)}\right)|V, F, \tilde{Y}\right) - \tau\right] - \right.$$

$$exp\left(\frac{y_i - \beta_0 - \beta_V'V_i - \beta_F'F_i}{exp(\tau)}\right) \cdot \mathbb{E}\left(\left(exp\left(-\frac{\beta_V'U_i}{exp(\tau)}\right)\right)|V, F, \tilde{Y}\right) \cdot$$

$$\frac{1}{M_{U_i}(\beta_V^+)}\ \Bigg]$$

$$\overset{(B.5),(B.6)}{=} \sum_{i=1}^{n}\left[\ \delta_i\left[\left(\frac{y_i - \beta_0 - \beta_V'V_i - \beta_F'F_i}{exp(\tau)}\right) - \tau\right] - exp\left(\frac{y_i - \beta_0 - \beta_V'V_i - \beta_F'F_i}{exp(\tau)}\right)\right]$$

$$= \sum_{i=1}^{n}\left[\ \delta_i\left[\left(\frac{y_i - X_i'\beta_X}{exp(\tau)}\right) - \tau\right] - exp\left(\frac{y_i - X_i'\beta_X}{exp(\tau)}\right)\right]$$

$$= l^X(t, X, \beta_X, \tau)$$

Given that U_i is independent of V_i, F_i, T_i and δ_i, $i = 1, \ldots n$, the following is used in the proof

$$\mathbb{E}\left(-\frac{\beta_V'U_i}{exp(\tau)}\ \bigg|\ V, F, \tilde{Y}\right) = \mathbb{E}\left(-\frac{\beta_V'U_i}{exp(\tau)}\right) = -\frac{\beta_V}{exp(\tau)} \cdot \mathbb{E}(U_i) = \beta_V^+ \cdot \mathbb{E}(U_i) = 0$$

$$(B.5)$$

$$\mathbb{E}\left(exp\left(-\frac{\beta'_V U_i}{exp(\tau)}\right)\ \bigg|\ V, F, \tilde{Y}\right) = \mathbb{E}\left(exp\left(-\frac{\beta'_V U_i}{exp(\tau)}\right)\right)$$
$$= \mathbb{E}\left(exp(\beta_V^+ U'_i)\right) = M_{U_i}(\beta_V^+),$$

(B.6)

with $\beta_V^+ = -\beta_V/exp(\tau) = -\beta_V/\nu$. Because F_i denotes error free variable(s), the moment generating function is set to 1, this means that

$$ln(M_{U_i}(\beta_X^+)) \overset{U_i \perp (V_i, F_i)}{=} ln(M_{U_i}(\beta_V^+) \cdot M_{U_i}(\beta_F^+))$$
$$= ln(M_{U_i}(\beta_V^+)) + ln(M_{U_i}(\beta_F^+)) \overset{M_{U_i}(\beta_F^+)=1}{=} ln(M_{U_i}(\beta_V^+)).$$

(B.7)

By the law of iterated expectation it follows that $\mathbb{E}(l^A_{corr}(t, A, \beta_X, \tau)|V, F, \tilde{Y}) = 0$ (cf. Equation (2.15)).

B.5. Weibull Model - Corrected Score Functions

In Appendix B.4 it was shown that the corrected log-likelihood from Equation (2.49) fulfils the condition of being an unbiased estimation equation. Condition (2.12) implies that the differentiation with respect to the parameters provides the according corrected score function(s). Here, the corrected score functions are the derivatives of $l^A_{corr}(\pi, A, \beta_X, \tau)$ with respect to β_X and τ. For β_X the corrected score function is derived as follows

$$\frac{\partial l^A_{corr}(t, A, \beta_X, \tau)}{\partial \beta_X}$$
$$= \sum_{i=1}^{n}\left[\delta_i\left(\frac{-A_i}{exp(\tau)}\right) - exp\left(\frac{y_i - \beta'_X A_i}{exp(\tau)} - ln(M_{U_i}(\beta_X^+))\right)\right.$$
$$\left.\left(\frac{-A'_i}{exp(\tau)} - \frac{\partial}{\partial \beta_X}ln(M_{U_i}(\beta_X^+))\right)\right]$$
$$= \sum_{i=1}^{n}\left[-\delta_i\left(\frac{A_i}{exp(\tau)}\right) + exp\left(\frac{y_i - \beta'_X A_i}{exp(\tau)} - ln(M_{U_i}(\beta_X^+))\right)\right.$$
$$\left.\left(\frac{A_i}{exp(\tau)} + \frac{\partial}{\partial \beta_X}ln(M_{U_i}(\beta_X^+))\right)\right]$$

(B.8)

For τ the corrected score function is derived as follows

$$
\frac{\partial l_{corr}^A(t, A, \beta_X, \tau)}{\partial \beta_X}
$$

$$
= \sum_{i=1}^{n} \left[\delta_i \left[-\left(\frac{y_i - \beta_X' A_i}{exp(\tau)} \right) - 1 \right] - exp\left(\frac{y_i - \beta_X' A_i}{exp(\tau)} - ln(M_{U_i}(\beta_X^+)) \right) \cdot \right.
$$

$$
\left. \left[-\frac{y_i - \beta_X' A_i}{exp(\tau)} - \frac{\partial}{\partial \tau} ln(M_{U_i}(\beta_X^+)) \right] \right] \tag{B.9}
$$

$$
= \sum_{i=1}^{n} \left[-\delta_i \left[1 + \left(\frac{y_i - \beta_X' A_i}{exp(\tau)} \right) \right] + exp\left(\frac{y_i - \beta_X' A_i}{exp(\tau)} - ln(M_{U_i}(\beta_X^+)) \right) \cdot \right.
$$

$$
\left. \left[\frac{y_i - \beta_X' A_i}{exp(\tau)} + \frac{\partial}{\partial \tau} ln(M_{U_i}(\beta_X^+)) \right] \right]
$$

with $(1/exp(\tau))' = (exp(-\tau))' = -exp(-\tau) = -(1/exp(\tau))$ and $(1/exp(\tau)^2)' = (exp(-2\tau))' = -2 \cdot exp(-2\tau) = -(2/exp(\tau)^2)$.

B.6. Weibull Model - Corrected Log-Likelihood with Interaction Term

Assuming the model equation

$$
\tilde{Y} \sim W + Z_1 + W \cdot Z, \tag{B.10}
$$

where $\tilde{Y}$ denotes the censored survival times, W the error-prone covariable and Z the partitioning variable. Here, a corrected log-likelihood has to be derived, which includes an adjustment for the main effect of the error-prone variable but also for the effect of the interaction term. In the following such a corrected log-likelihood is derived for the Weibull model, which fulfils the condition (2.13) of being an unbiased estimation equation. Furthermore, the corrected score functions are derived from the corrected log-likelihood for normal homoscedastic errors.

Given the corrected log-likelihood of the Weibull model from Equation (2.49) with $\beta_X' A_i = \beta_0 + \beta_V' W_i + \beta_Z' Z_i + \beta_{VZ}' W_i \cdot Z_i$ and accordingly $\beta_X' X_i = \beta_0 + \beta_V' V_i + \beta_Z' Z_i + \beta_{VZ}' V_i \cdot Z_i$. At first, it has to be shown that $\mathbb{E}(l_{corr}^A(t, A, \beta_X, \tau)|V, Z, \tilde{Y}) = l^X(t, X, \beta_X, \tau)$.

$$\mathbb{E}(l_{corr}^A(t, A, \beta_X, \tau)|V, Z, \tilde{Y})$$

$$= \mathbb{E}\left(\sum_{i=1}^{n}\left[\delta_i\left[\left(\frac{y_i - \beta_X' A_i}{exp(\tau)}\right) - \tau\right] - exp\left(\frac{y_i - \beta_X' A_i}{exp(\tau)} - ln(M_{U_i}(a_i))\right)\right]\middle| V, Z, \tilde{Y}\right)$$

$$= \mathbb{E}\left(\sum_{i=1}^{n}\left[\delta_i\left[\left(\frac{y_i - (\beta_0 + \beta_V' W_i + \beta_Z' Z_i + \beta_{VZ}' W_i \cdot Z_i)}{exp(\tau)}\right) - \tau\right] - exp\left(\frac{y_i - (\beta_0 + \beta_V' W_i + \beta_Z' Z_i + \beta_{VZ}' W_i \cdot Z_i)}{exp(\tau)} - ln(M_{U_i}(a_i))\right)\right]\middle| V, Z, \tilde{Y}\right)$$

$$= \mathbb{E}\left(\sum_{i=1}^{n}\left[\delta_i\left[\left(\frac{y_i - (\beta_0 + \beta_V'(V_i + U_i) + \beta_Z' Z_i + \beta_{VZ}'(V_i + U_i) \cdot Z_i)}{exp(\tau)}\right) - \tau\right] - exp\left(\frac{y_i - (\beta_0 + \beta_V'(V_i + U_i) + \beta_Z' Z_i + \beta_{VZ}'(V_i + U_i) \cdot Z_i)}{exp(\tau)} - ln(M_{U_i}(a_i))\right)\right]\middle| V, Z, \tilde{Y}\right)$$

$$= \mathbb{E}\left(\sum_{i=1}^{n}\left[\delta_i\left[\left(\frac{y_i - (\beta_0 + \beta_V' V_i + \beta_V' U_i + \beta_Z' Z_i + \beta_{VZ}' V_i \cdot Z_i + \beta_{VZ}' U_i \cdot Z_i)}{exp(\tau)}\right) - \tau\right] - exp\left(\frac{y_i - (\beta_0 + \beta_V' V_i + \beta_V' U_i + \beta_Z' Z_i + \beta_{VZ}' V_i \cdot Z_i + \beta_{VZ}' U_i \cdot Z_i)}{exp(\tau)} - ln(M_{U_i}(a_i))\right)\right]\middle| V, Z, \tilde{Y}\right)$$

$$= \mathbb{E}\left(\sum_{i=1}^{n}\left[\delta_i\left(\left(\frac{y_i}{exp(\tau)} - \frac{\beta_0}{exp(\tau)} - \frac{\beta_V' V_i}{exp(\tau)} - \frac{\beta_V' U_i}{exp(\tau)} - \frac{\beta_Z' Z_i}{exp(\tau)} - \frac{\beta_{VZ}' V_i \cdot Z_i}{exp(\tau)} - \frac{\beta_{VZ}' U_i \cdot Z_i}{exp(\tau)}\right) - \tau\right) - \left(exp\left(\frac{y_i}{exp(\tau)}\right) \cdot exp\left(-\frac{\beta_0}{exp(\tau)}\right) \cdot exp\left(-\frac{\beta_V' V_i}{exp(\tau)}\right) \cdot exp\left(-\frac{\beta_V' U_i}{exp(\tau)}\right) \cdot exp\left(-\frac{\beta_Z' Z_i}{exp(\tau)}\right) \cdot exp\left(-\frac{\beta_{VZ}' V_i \cdot Z_i}{exp(\tau)}\right) \cdot exp\left(-\frac{\beta_{VZ}' U_i \cdot Z_i}{exp(\tau)}\right) \cdot exp(-ln(M_{U_i}(a_i)))\right)\right]\middle| V, Z, \tilde{Y}\right)$$

$$= \mathbb{E}\left(\sum_{i=1}^{n}\left[\delta_i\left(\left(\frac{y_i}{exp(\tau)} - \frac{\beta_0}{exp(\tau)} - \frac{\beta_V' V_i}{exp(\tau)} - \frac{\beta_Z' Z_i}{exp(\tau)} - \frac{\beta_{VZ}' V_i \cdot Z_i}{exp(\tau)} - \right.\right.\right.$$

$$\frac{(\beta_V' + \beta_{VZ}' \cdot Z_i)U_i}{exp(\tau)} \Bigg) - \tau \Bigg) - \Bigg(exp\left(\frac{y_i}{exp(\tau)}\right) \cdot exp\left(-\frac{\beta_0}{exp(\tau)}\right) \cdot$$

$$exp\left(-\frac{\beta_V' V_i}{exp(\tau)}\right) \cdot exp\left(-\frac{\beta_Z' Z_i}{exp(\tau)}\right) \cdot exp\left(-\frac{\beta_{VZ}' V_i \cdot Z_i}{exp(\tau)}\right) \cdot$$

$$exp\left(-\frac{(\beta_V' + \beta_{VZ}' \cdot Z_i)U_i}{exp(\tau)}\right) \cdot exp(-ln(M_{U_i}(a_i))) \Bigg) \Bigg] \Bigg| V, Z, \tilde{Y} \Bigg)$$

$$= \sum_{i=1}^{n} \Bigg[\delta_i \Bigg(\Bigg(\frac{y_i}{exp(\tau)} - \frac{\beta_0}{exp(\tau)} - \frac{\beta_V' V_i}{exp(\tau)} - \frac{\beta_Z' Z_i}{exp(\tau)} - \frac{\beta_{VZ}' V_i \cdot Z_i}{exp(\tau)} +$$

$$\mathbb{E}\left(-\frac{(\beta_V' + \beta_{VZ}' \cdot Z_i)U_i}{exp(\tau)} \Bigg| V, Z, \tilde{Y} \right) \Bigg) - \tau \Bigg) - \Bigg(exp\left(\frac{y_i}{exp(\tau)}\right) \cdot$$

$$exp\left(-\frac{\beta_0}{exp(\tau)}\right) \cdot exp\left(-\frac{\beta_V' V_i}{exp(\tau)}\right) \cdot exp\left(-\frac{\beta_Z' Z_i}{exp(\tau)}\right) \cdot exp\left(-\frac{\beta_{VZ}' V_i \cdot Z_i}{exp(\tau)}\right) \cdot$$

$$\mathbb{E}\left(exp\left(-\frac{(\beta_V' + \beta_{VZ}' \cdot Z_i)U_i}{exp(\tau)}\right) \Bigg| V, Z, \tilde{Y} \right) \cdot \frac{1}{M_{U_i}(a_i)} \Bigg) \Bigg]$$

$$\overset{(B.11)(B.12)}{=} \sum_{i=1}^{n} \Bigg[\delta_i \Bigg(\Bigg(\frac{y_i}{exp(\tau)} - \frac{\beta_0}{exp(\tau)} - \frac{\beta_V' V_i}{exp(\tau)} - \frac{\beta_Z' Z_i}{exp(\tau)} - \frac{\beta_{VZ}' V_i \cdot Z_i}{exp(\tau)} \Bigg) - \tau \Bigg)$$

$$- \Bigg(exp\left(\frac{y_i}{exp(\tau)}\right) \cdot exp\left(-\frac{\beta_0}{exp(\tau)}\right) \cdot exp\left(-\frac{\beta_V' V_i}{exp(\tau)}\right) \cdot$$

$$exp\left(-\frac{\beta_Z' Z_i}{exp(\tau)}\right) \cdot exp\left(-\frac{\beta_{VZ}' V_i \cdot Z_i}{exp(\tau)}\right) \Bigg) \Bigg]$$

$$= \sum_{i=1}^{n} \Bigg[\delta_i \Bigg(\Bigg(\frac{y_i}{exp(\tau)} - \frac{\beta_X' X_i}{exp(\tau)} \Bigg) - \tau \Bigg) - exp\left(\frac{y_i}{exp(\tau)} - \frac{\beta_X' X_i}{exp(\tau)}\right) \Bigg]$$

$$= \sum_{i=1}^{n} \Bigg[\delta_i \Bigg(\Bigg(\frac{y_i - \beta_X' X_i}{exp(\tau)} \Bigg) - \tau \Bigg) - exp\left(\frac{y_i - \beta_X' X_i}{exp(\tau)}\right) \Bigg]$$

$$= l^X(t, X, \beta_X, \tau)$$

Given that U_i is independent of V_i, Z_i, T_i and δ_i, $i = 1, \ldots n$, the following is used in the proof

$$\mathbb{E}\left(-\frac{(\beta_V' + \beta_{VZ}' \cdot Z_i)U_i}{exp(\tau)} \Bigg| V, Z, \tilde{Y} \right) = \mathbb{E}\left(-\frac{(\beta_V' + \beta_{VZ}' \cdot Z_i)U_i}{exp(\tau)} \right)$$

$$= -\frac{(\beta_V' + \beta_{VZ}' \cdot Z_i)}{exp(\tau)} \cdot \mathbb{E}(U_i) = 0 \qquad \text{(B.11)}$$

$$\mathbb{E}\left(exp\left(-\frac{(\beta_V' + \beta_{VZ}' \cdot Z_i)U_i}{exp(\tau)}\right)\ \middle|\ V, Z, \tilde{Y}\right) = \mathbb{E}\left(exp\left(-\frac{(\beta_V' + \beta_{VZ}' \cdot Z_i)U_i}{exp(\tau)}\right)\right)$$

$$= \mathbb{E}\left(exp\left(-\frac{\beta_V'}{exp(\tau)} - \frac{\beta_{VZ}' \cdot Z_i}{exp(\tau)}\right)U_i\right) = \mathbb{E}(exp((\underbrace{\beta_V^{+\prime} + \beta_{VZ}^{+\prime} \cdot Z_i}_{:=a_i'})U_i)) = M_{U_i}(a_i),$$

$$\text{(B.12)}$$

with $\beta_V^+ = -\beta_V/exp(\tau) = -\beta_V/\nu$ and $\beta_{VZ}^+ = -\beta_{VZ}/exp(\tau) = -\beta_{VZ}/\nu$. In the case of normal homoscedastic errors the moment generating function $M_{U_i}(a_i)$, with $a_i = \beta_V^+ + \beta_{VZ}^+ \cdot Z_i$, can be specified further

$$M_U((\beta_V^+ + \beta_{VZ}^+ \cdot Z_i)) = exp\left(\frac{1}{2}(\beta_V^+ + \beta_{VZ}^+ \cdot Z_i)'\Sigma_U(\beta_V^+ + \beta_{VZ}^+ \cdot Z_i)\right) \quad \text{(B.13)}$$

$$= exp\left(\frac{(\beta_V + \beta_{VZ} \cdot Z_i)'\Sigma_U(\beta_V + \beta_{VZ} \cdot Z_i)}{2 \cdot exp(\tau)^2}\right). \quad \text{(B.14)}$$

Furthermore,

$$ln(M_U((\beta_V^+ + \beta_{VZ}^+ \cdot Z_i))) = \frac{(\beta_V + \beta_{VZ} \cdot Z_i)'\Sigma_U(\beta_V + \beta_{VZ} \cdot Z_i)}{2 \cdot exp(\tau)^2} \quad \text{(B.15)}$$

$$\frac{\partial}{\partial \beta_X}ln(M_U((\beta_V^+ + \beta_{VZ}^+ \cdot Z_i))) = \begin{pmatrix} \frac{\partial}{\partial \beta_0}ln(M_U((\beta_V^+ + \beta_{VZ}^+ \cdot Z_i))) \\ \frac{\partial}{\partial \beta_V}ln(M_U((\beta_V^+ + \beta_{VZ}^+ \cdot Z_i))) \\ \frac{\partial}{\partial \beta_{VZ}}ln(M_U((\beta_V^+ + \beta_{VZ}^+ \cdot Z_i))) \\ \frac{\partial}{\partial \beta_Z}ln(M_U((\beta_V^+ + \beta_{VZ}^+ \cdot Z_i))) \end{pmatrix}$$
$$= \begin{pmatrix} 0 \\ \frac{(\beta_V + \beta_{VZ}' \cdot Z_i)\Sigma_U}{exp(\tau)^2} \\ \frac{(\beta_{VZ}Z_i'Z_i + \beta_V' \cdot Z_i)\Sigma_U}{exp(\tau)^2} \\ 0 \end{pmatrix} \quad \text{(B.16)}$$

$$\frac{\partial}{\partial \tau}ln(M_U((\beta_V^+ + \beta_{VZ}^+ \cdot Z_i))) = -\frac{(\beta_V + \beta_{VZ} \cdot Z_i)'\Sigma_U(\beta_V + \beta_{VZ} \cdot Z_i)}{exp(\tau)^2}. \quad \text{(B.17)}$$

with $(\beta_V + \beta_{VZ} \cdot Z_i)'(\beta_V + \beta_{VZ} \cdot Z_i) = \beta_V'\beta_V + \beta_{VZ}'Z_i'Z_i\beta_{VZ} + 2\beta_{VZ}'Z_i'\beta_V$. Substituting Equations (B.15) – (B.17) in (2.49), (2.50) and (2.51) leads to the corrected log-likelihood

$$
\begin{aligned}
l_{corr}^{A}(t, A, \beta_X, \tau) = \sum_{i=1}^{n} & \Bigg[\delta_i \left[\left(\frac{y_i - \beta_X' A_i}{exp(\tau)} \right) - \tau \right] - exp \left(\frac{y_i - \beta_X' A_i}{exp(\tau)} - \right. \\
& \left. \frac{(\beta_V + \beta_{VZ} \cdot Z_i)' \Sigma_U (\beta_V + \beta_{VZ} \cdot Z_i)}{2 \cdot exp(\tau)^2} \right) \Bigg],
\end{aligned}
\tag{B.18}
$$

to the corrected score function of β_X

$$
\begin{aligned}
s_{corr_{\beta_X}}^{A}(t, A, \beta_X, \tau) = \sum_{i=1}^{n} & \Bigg[-\delta_i \left(\frac{A_i}{exp(\tau)} \right) + \\
& exp \left(\frac{y_i - \beta_X' A_i}{exp(\tau)} - \frac{(\beta_V + \beta_{VZ} \cdot Z_i)' \Sigma_U (\beta_V + \beta_{VZ} \cdot Z_i)}{2 \cdot exp(\tau)^2} \right) \cdot \\
& \left(\frac{A_i}{exp(\tau)} + \frac{\partial}{\partial \beta_X} ln(M_U((\beta_V + \beta_{VZ} \cdot Z_i))) \right) \Bigg] \\
= \frac{1}{exp(\tau)} \sum_{i=1}^{n} & \Bigg[exp \left(\frac{y_i - \beta_X' A_i}{exp(\tau)} - \frac{(\beta_V + \beta_{VZ} \cdot Z_i)' \Sigma_U (\beta_V + \beta_{VZ} \cdot Z_i)}{2 \cdot exp(\tau)^2} \right) \cdot \\
& \left(\begin{pmatrix} 1 \\ W_i \\ W_i \cdot Z_i \\ Z_i \end{pmatrix} + \begin{pmatrix} 0 \\ \frac{(\beta_V + \beta_{VZ}' \cdot Z_i) \Sigma_U}{exp(\tau)} \\ \frac{(\beta_{VZ} Z_i' Z_i + \beta_V \cdot Z_i) \Sigma_U}{exp(\tau)} \\ 0 \end{pmatrix} \right) - \delta_i A_i \Bigg],
\end{aligned}
\tag{B.19}
$$

and to the corrected score function of τ

$$
\begin{aligned}
s_{corr_{\tau}}^{A}(t, A, \beta_X, \tau) = \sum_{i=1}^{n} & \Bigg[-\delta_i \left[1 + \left(\frac{y_i - \beta_X' A_i}{exp(\tau)} \right) \right] + \\
& exp \left(\frac{y_i - \beta_X' A_i}{exp(\tau)} - \frac{(\beta_V + \beta_{VZ} \cdot Z_i)' \Sigma_U (\beta_V + \beta_{VZ} \cdot Z_i)}{2 \cdot exp(\tau)^2} \right) \cdot \\
& \left[\frac{y_i - \beta_X' A_i}{exp(\tau)} - \frac{(\beta_V + \beta_{VZ} \cdot Z_i)' \Sigma_U (\beta_V + \beta_{VZ} \cdot Z_i)}{exp(\tau)^2} \right] \Bigg].
\end{aligned}
\tag{B.20}
$$

B.7. Generating Failure Times

Assuming the parameterisation of the Weibull distribution as in Section 2.1.3. Then $F(T) = 1 - exp(-(b \cdot T)^a)$ and $S(T) = exp(-(b \cdot T)^a)$. The failure time T is derived via the distribution function $F(T)$. If T is a random number, then $D = F(T)$ is uniformly distributed in $[0, 1]$. If $D \sim Unif(0, 1)$, then $(1 - D) \sim Unif(0, 1)$ holds, too (cf. Bender et al., 2005).

With $D \sim Unif(0,1)$ and $b = exp(-\beta_X' X)$, $a = 1/\nu$ and $\tau = ln(\nu)$

$$D = exp(-(b \cdot t)^a)$$
$$= exp(-(exp(-\beta_X' X) \cdot t)^{1/\nu})$$
$$= exp\left(-exp\left(-\frac{\beta_X' X}{\nu}\right) \cdot t^{1/\nu}\right)$$

$$\Leftrightarrow$$

$$-ln(D) = exp\left(-\frac{\beta_X' X}{\nu}\right) \cdot t^{1/\nu}$$

$$-ln(D) \cdot exp\left(\frac{\beta_X' X}{\nu}\right) = t^{1/\nu}$$

$$\rightarrow T = \left(-log(D) \cdot exp\left(\frac{\beta_X' X}{\nu}\right)\right)^\nu$$

$$\rightarrow T = \left(-log(D) \cdot exp\left(\frac{\beta_X' X}{exp(\tau)}\right)\right)^{exp(\tau)}$$

B.8. Mean Expected Failure Time

Considering the mean expected failure time is useful to see how the differences between the resulting parameter estimates affect the expected failure time. Assuming the model equation of the Weibull model

$$ln(T_i) = \beta_X' X_i + \nu \cdot \epsilon$$

from Equation (2.43). Solving this equation for T_i results in

$$T_i = exp(\beta_X' X_i) \cdot exp(\nu \cdot \epsilon).$$

Taking the conditional expectation and a few transformations leads to

$$\mathbb{E}(T_i | X_i) = exp(\beta_X' X_i) \cdot \mathbb{E}(exp(\nu \cdot \epsilon) | X_i)$$
$$= exp(\beta_X' X_i) \cdot \Gamma\left(\frac{1 + (1/\nu)}{1/\nu}\right)$$
$$= exp(\beta_X' X_i) \cdot \Gamma(\nu + 1)$$
$$= exp(\beta_X' X_i) \cdot \Gamma(exp(\tau) + 1)$$

Substituting the mean value of the covariable(s) $\bar{X}$ and the estimated model parameters lead to an estimation of the mean expected failure time

$$\widehat{\mathbb{E}(T|X)} = exp(\hat{\beta}'_X \bar{X})\Gamma(exp(\hat{\tau}) + 1).$$

C. Results of the Simulation Study

The simulation study consists of three parts. In the following only selected results are presented. In Appendix C.1 and C.2 the results are presented for the separate consideration of the new implemented `fit` function `SurvRegcorr@fit()` including only W as well as including W and F, respectively. In Appendix C.3 selected results of the detection rate for the true underlying single tree structure are shown as well as the results of the parameter estimation in the terminal nodes. In Appendix C.4 the detection rates for multiple structural changes are presented as well as the model summaries including the parameter estimates for one selected example. In Appendix C.5 the results of the prediction error are shown for the global model and the MOB.

C.1. Check the `fit` function - only W

C.1.1. `beta.true` = -0.2, `tau.true` = -0.3, `prob.cens` = 35% and $V \sim N(0, 1)$

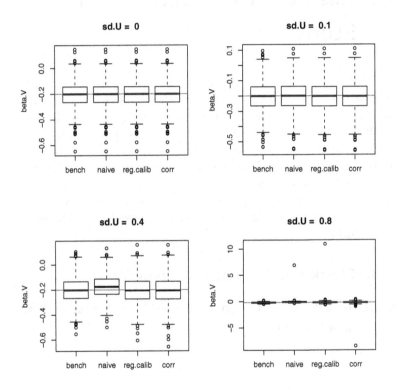

Figure C.1.: Boxplot for β_V with beta.true = -0.2, tau.true = -0.3, prob.cens = 35%, $V \sim N(0,1)$, size = 100

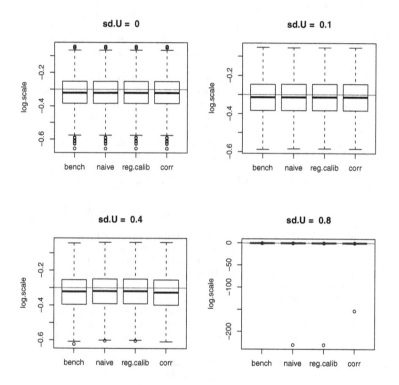

Figure C.2.: Boxplot for τ with beta.true = -0.2, tau.true = -0.3, prob.cens = 35%, $V \sim N(0,1)$, size = 100

	$\hat{\bar{\beta}}_V$	$med(\hat{\beta}_V)$	$sd(\hat{\beta}_V)$	$\overline{sd(\hat{\beta}_V)}$	$\% \in$ CI	$\widehat{MSE}$	$\widehat{\mathbb{E}(T)}$
sd.U $= 0$							
benchmark	-0.202	-0.200	0.093	0.094	96.600	0.009	0.916
naive	-0.202	-0.200	0.093	0.094	96.600	0.009	0.916
reg.calib	-0.202	-0.200	0.093	0.094	96.600	0.009	0.916
corr	-0.202	-0.200	0.093	0.092	95.400	0.009	0.916
sd.U $= 0.1$							
benchmark	-0.202	-0.201	0.093	0.095	95.000	0.009	0.918
naive	-0.201	-0.200	0.093	0.094	95.300	0.009	0.918
reg.calib	-0.203	-0.202	0.094	0.095	95.500	0.009	0.918
corr	-0.203	-0.202	0.094	0.094	94.400	0.009	0.918
sd.U $= 0.4$							
benchmark	-0.202	-0.203	0.098	0.094	94.500	0.010	0.917
naive	-0.174	-0.176	0.091	0.088	91.900	0.009	0.918
reg.calib	-0.203	-0.205	0.107	0.103	94.400	0.011	0.918
corr	-0.205	-0.206	0.109	0.102	93.300	0.012	0.917
sd.U $= 0.8$							
benchmark	-0.203	-0.198	0.095	0.095	95.600	0.009	0.916
naive	-0.116	-0.123	0.233	0.074	80.700	0.062	0.919
reg.calib	-0.193	-0.200	0.374	0.124	94.600	0.140	0.919
corr	-0.223	-0.204	0.299	75512	95.775	0.090	0.916

	$\hat{\bar{\tau}}$	$med(\hat{\tau})$	$sd(\hat{\tau})$	$\overline{sd(\hat{\tau})}$	$\% \in$ CI	$\widehat{MSE}$	#NA
sd.U $= 0$							
benchmark	-0.320	-0.321	0.099	0.098	94.400	0.010	0
naive	-0.320	-0.321	0.099	0.098	94.400	0.010	0
reg.calib	-0.320	-0.321	0.099	0.098	94.400	0.010	0
corr	-0.320	-0.321	0.099	0.097	93.400	0.010	0
sd.U $= 0.1$							
benchmark	-0.316	-0.314	0.101	0.098	94.200	0.010	0
naive	-0.316	-0.314	0.101	0.098	94.100	0.010	0
reg.calib	-0.316	-0.314	0.101	0.098	94.100	0.010	0
corr	-0.316	-0.314	0.101	0.097	93.200	0.010	0
sd.U $= 0.4$							
benchmark	-0.323	-0.321	0.101	0.098	93.400	0.011	0
naive	-0.319	-0.319	0.102	0.098	93.300	0.011	0
reg.calib	-0.319	-0.319	0.102	0.098	93.300	0.011	0
corr	-0.325	-0.326	0.103	0.099	92.300	0.011	0
sd.U $= 0.8$							
benchmark	-0.318	-0.313	0.100	0.098	93.700	0.010	0
naive	-0.538	-0.303	7.285	0.098	94.700	53.079	0
reg.calib	-0.538	-0.303	7.285	0.098	94.700	53.079	0
corr	-0.480	-0.319	4.868	0.104	93.964	23.709	6

Table C.1.: Results for β_V and τ with `beta.true` = -0.2, `tau.true` = -0.3, `prob.cens` = 35%, $V \sim N(0,1)$ and `size` = 100

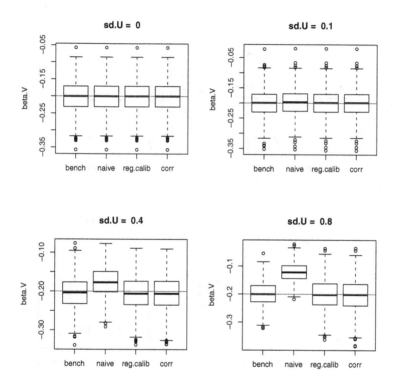

Figure C.3.: Boxplot for β_V with beta.true = -0.2, tau.true = -0.3, prob.cens = 35%, $V \sim N(0,1)$, size = 500

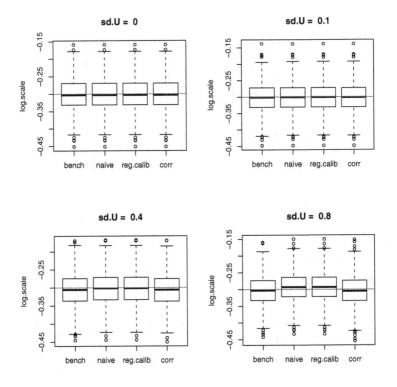

Figure C.4.: Boxplot for τ with beta.true = -0.2, tau.true = -0.3, prob.cens = 35%, $V \sim N(0, 1)$, size = 500

	$\bar{\hat{\beta}}_V$	$med(\hat{\beta}_V)$	$sd(\hat{\beta}_V)$	$\overline{sd(\hat{\beta}_V)}$	$\% \in$ CI	$\widehat{MSE}$	$\widehat{\mathbb{E}(T)}$
sd.U = 0							
benchmark	-0.201	-0.200	0.045	0.042	92.900	0.002	0.917
naive	-0.201	-0.200	0.045	0.042	92.900	0.002	0.917
reg.calib	-0.201	-0.200	0.045	0.042	92.900	0.002	0.917
corr	-0.201	-0.200	0.045	0.042	92.200	0.002	0.917
sd.U = 0.1							
benchmark	-0.200	-0.199	0.043	0.042	94.700	0.002	0.917
naive	-0.198	-0.197	0.043	0.042	94.200	0.002	0.917
reg.calib	-0.200	-0.199	0.043	0.042	94.300	0.002	0.917
corr	-0.200	-0.199	0.044	0.042	94.200	0.002	0.917
sd.U = 0.4							
benchmark	-0.204	-0.204	0.041	0.042	95.700	0.002	0.917
naive	-0.176	-0.177	0.038	0.039	90.400	0.002	0.917
reg.calib	-0.204	-0.206	0.044	0.045	95.700	0.002	0.917
corr	-0.205	-0.206	0.045	0.045	95.300	0.002	0.917
sd.U = 0.8							
benchmark	-0.200	-0.200	0.042	0.042	94.800	0.002	0.917
naive	-0.122	-0.122	0.033	0.033	33.500	0.007	0.919
reg.calib	-0.200	-0.202	0.055	0.054	94.100	0.003	0.919
corr	-0.203	-0.201	0.057	0.056	94.200	0.003	0.917

	$\bar{\hat{\tau}}$	$med(\hat{\tau})$	$sd(\hat{\tau})$	$\overline{sd(\hat{\tau})}$	$\% \in$ CI	$\widehat{MSE}$	#NA
sd.U = 0							
benchmark	-0.302	-0.303	0.045	0.044	94.500	0.002	0
naive	-0.302	-0.303	0.045	0.044	94.500	0.002	0
reg.calib	-0.302	-0.303	0.045	0.044	94.500	0.002	0
corr	-0.302	-0.303	0.045	0.044	94.400	0.002	0
sd.U = 0.1							
benchmark	-0.301	-0.301	0.043	0.044	95.500	0.002	0
naive	-0.301	-0.301	0.043	0.044	95.500	0.002	0
reg.calib	-0.301	-0.301	0.043	0.044	95.500	0.002	0
corr	-0.301	-0.301	0.043	0.044	95.300	0.002	0
sd.U = 0.4							
benchmark	-0.305	-0.305	0.043	0.044	95.800	0.002	0
naive	-0.301	-0.301	0.043	0.044	95.300	0.002	0
reg.calib	-0.301	-0.301	0.043	0.044	95.300	0.002	0
corr	-0.306	-0.306	0.044	0.044	95.300	0.002	0
sd.U = 0.8							
benchmark	-0.303	-0.303	0.044	0.044	93.900	0.002	0
naive	-0.293	-0.294	0.044	0.044	94.000	0.002	0
reg.calib	-0.293	-0.294	0.044	0.044	94.000	0.002	0
corr	-0.305	-0.305	0.045	0.045	94.200	0.002	0

Table C.2.: Results for β_V and τ with beta.true = -0.2, tau.true = -0.3, prob.cens = 35%, $V \sim N(0,1)$ and size = 500

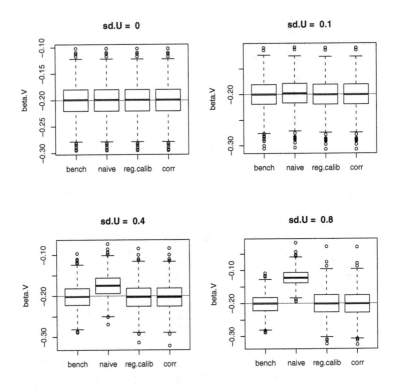

Figure C.5.: Boxplot for β_V with beta.true = -0.2, tau.true = -0.3, prob.cens = 35%, $V \sim N(0,1)$, size = 1000

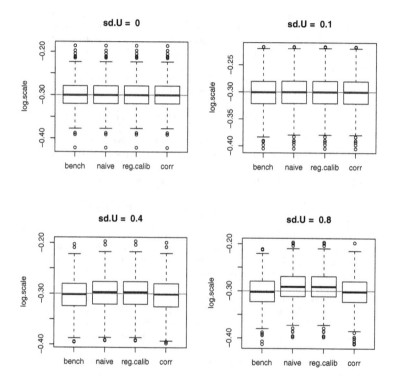

Figure C.6.: Boxplot for τ with `beta.true` = -0.2, `tau.true` = -0.3, `prob.cens` = 35%, $V \sim N(0,1)$, `size` = 1000

	$\bar{\hat{\beta}}_V$	$med(\hat{\beta}_V)$	$sd(\hat{\beta}_V)$	$\overline{sd(\hat{\beta}_V)}$	% $\in$ CI	$\widehat{MSE}$	$\widehat{\mathbb{E}(T)}$
sd.U = 0							
benchmark	-0.200	-0.199	0.031	0.030	93.200	0.001	0.917
naive	-0.200	-0.199	0.031	0.030	93.200	0.001	0.917
reg.calib	-0.200	-0.199	0.031	0.030	93.200	0.001	0.917
corr	-0.200	-0.199	0.031	0.030	93.100	0.001	0.917
sd.U = 0.1							
benchmark	-0.201	-0.200	0.030	0.030	94.700	0.001	0.917
naive	-0.199	-0.198	0.030	0.029	94.700	0.001	0.917
reg.calib	-0.201	-0.200	0.030	0.030	94.600	0.001	0.917
corr	-0.201	-0.200	0.030	0.030	94.700	0.001	0.917
sd.U = 0.4							
benchmark	-0.202	-0.201	0.030	0.029	93.900	0.001	0.917
naive	-0.174	-0.175	0.028	0.027	83.400	0.001	0.917
reg.calib	-0.202	-0.202	0.032	0.032	94.800	0.001	0.917
corr	-0.203	-0.203	0.032	0.032	94.700	0.001	0.917
sd.U = 0.8							
benchmark	-0.202	-0.201	0.030	0.030	95.300	0.001	0.917
naive	-0.122	-0.123	0.024	0.023	8.800	0.007	0.919
reg.calib	-0.201	-0.201	0.040	0.038	94.100	0.002	0.918
corr	-0.202	-0.202	0.041	0.040	94.700	0.002	0.917

	$\bar{\hat{\tau}}$	$med(\hat{\tau})$	$sd(\hat{\tau})$	$\overline{sd(\hat{\tau})}$	% $\in$ CI	$\widehat{MSE}$	#NA
sd.U = 0							
benchmark	-0.300	-0.300	0.030	0.031	96.000	0.001	0
naive	-0.300	-0.300	0.030	0.031	96.000	0.001	0
reg.calib	-0.300	-0.300	0.030	0.031	96.000	0.001	0
corr	-0.300	-0.300	0.030	0.031	96.000	0.001	0
sd.U = 0.1							
benchmark	-0.301	-0.300	0.030	0.031	95.900	0.001	0
naive	-0.301	-0.300	0.030	0.031	95.800	0.001	0
reg.calib	-0.301	-0.300	0.030	0.031	95.800	0.001	0
corr	-0.301	-0.300	0.030	0.031	95.600	0.001	0
sd.U = 0.4							
benchmark	-0.302	-0.301	0.032	0.031	94.100	0.001	0
naive	-0.298	-0.297	0.032	0.031	94.500	0.001	0
reg.calib	-0.298	-0.297	0.032	0.031	94.500	0.001	0
corr	-0.302	-0.301	0.032	0.031	93.800	0.001	0
sd.U = 0.8							
benchmark	-0.302	-0.302	0.031	0.031	94.900	0.001	0
naive	-0.291	-0.291	0.031	0.031	94.200	0.001	0
reg.calib	-0.291	-0.291	0.031	0.031	94.200	0.001	0
corr	-0.302	-0.302	0.032	0.032	94.600	0.001	0

Table C.3.: Results for β_V and τ with beta.true = -0.2, tau.true = -0.3, prob.cens = 35%, $V \sim N(0,1)$ and size = 1000

C.1.2. `beta.true` = **-0.2**, `tau.true` = **-0.3**, `prob.cens` = **35%** and $V \sim Unif(0, \sqrt{12})$

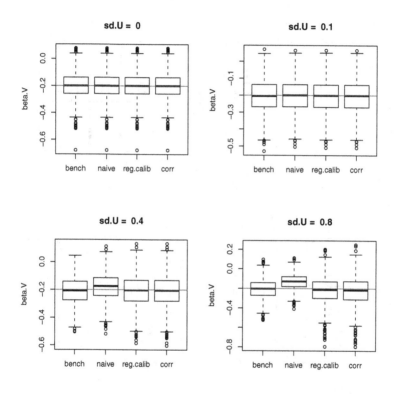

Figure C.7.: Boxplot for β_V with `beta.true` = -0.2, `tau.true` = -0.3, `prob.cens` = 35%, $V \sim Unif(0, \sqrt{12})$, `size` = 100

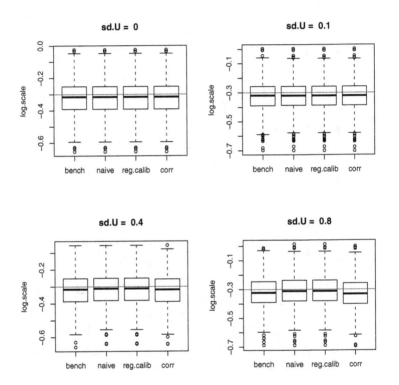

Figure C.8.: Boxplot for τ with beta.true = -0.2, tau.true = -0.3, prob.cens = 35%, $V \sim Unif(0, \sqrt{12})$, size = 100

	$\bar{\hat{\beta}}_V$	$med(\hat{\beta}_V)$	$sd(\hat{\beta}_V)$	$\overline{sd(\hat{\beta}_V)}$	$\% \in$ CI	$\widehat{MSE}$	$\widehat{\mathbb{E}(T)}$
sd.U = 0							
benchmark	-0.199	-0.199	0.095	0.093	94.200	0.009	0.658
naive	-0.199	-0.199	0.095	0.093	94.200	0.009	0.658
reg.calib	-0.199	-0.199	0.095	0.093	94.200	0.009	0.658
corr	-0.199	-0.199	0.095	0.092	94.100	0.009	0.658
sd.U = 0.1							
benchmark	-0.203	-0.205	0.096	0.093	93.400	0.009	0.654
naive	-0.201	-0.200	0.095	0.092	93.500	0.009	0.656
reg.calib	-0.203	-0.202	0.096	0.093	93.600	0.009	0.654
corr	-0.203	-0.202	0.096	0.092	93.400	0.009	0.654
sd.U = 0.4							
benchmark	-0.207	-0.207	0.098	0.093	94.000	0.010	0.650
naive	-0.180	-0.174	0.094	0.087	92.700	0.009	0.680
reg.calib	-0.209	-0.203	0.109	0.101	93.800	0.012	0.650
corr	-0.211	-0.204	0.111	0.101	93.200	0.012	0.648
sd.U = 0.8							
benchmark	-0.206	-0.203	0.096	0.094	94.500	0.009	0.651
naive	-0.129	-0.128	0.078	0.074	80.900	0.011	0.741
reg.calib	-0.218	-0.212	0.137	0.125	93.000	0.019	0.647
corr	-0.226	-0.217	0.148	0.140	95.846	0.023	0.640

	$\bar{\hat{\tau}}$	$med(\hat{\tau})$	$sd(\hat{\tau})$	$\overline{sd(\hat{\tau})}$	$\% \in$ CI	$\widehat{MSE}$	#NA
sd.U = 0							
benchmark	-0.319	-0.316	0.101	0.098	94.600	0.010	0
naive	-0.319	-0.316	0.101	0.098	94.600	0.010	0
reg.calib	-0.319	-0.316	0.101	0.098	94.600	0.010	0
corr	-0.319	-0.316	0.101	0.097	93.800	0.010	0
sd.U = 0.1							
benchmark	-0.324	-0.319	0.103	0.098	93.700	0.011	0
naive	-0.323	-0.320	0.103	0.098	93.500	0.011	0
reg.calib	-0.323	-0.320	0.103	0.098	93.500	0.011	0
corr	-0.324	-0.321	0.103	0.098	92.200	0.011	0
sd.U = 0.4							
benchmark	-0.320	-0.316	0.096	0.098	95.000	0.010	0
naive	-0.316	-0.311	0.096	0.098	95.300	0.009	0
reg.calib	-0.316	-0.311	0.096	0.098	95.300	0.009	0
corr	-0.321	-0.317	0.097	0.098	94.200	0.010	0
sd.U = 0.8							
benchmark	-0.318	-0.323	0.105	0.098	93.200	0.011	0
naive	-0.308	-0.312	0.105	0.098	93.400	0.011	0
reg.calib	-0.308	-0.312	0.105	0.098	93.400	0.011	0
corr	-0.329	-0.332	0.109	0.105	93.313	0.013	13

Table C.4.: Results for β_V and τ with `beta.true` = -0.2, `tau.true` = -0.3, `prob.cens` = 35%, $V \sim Unif(0, \sqrt{12})$ and `size` = 100

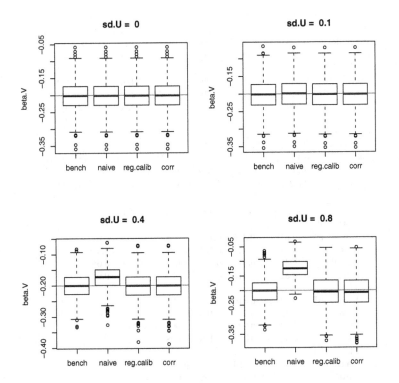

Figure C.9.: Boxplot for β_V with beta.true = -0.2, tau.true = -0.3, prob.cens = 35%, $V \sim Unif(0, \sqrt{12})$, size = 500

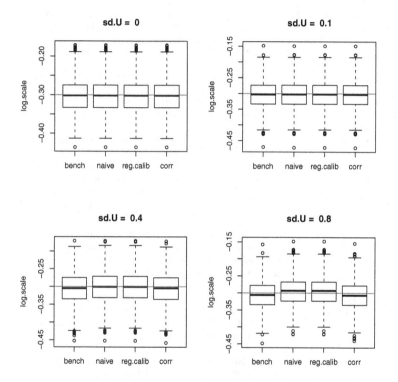

Figure C.10.: Boxplot for τ with beta.true = -0.2, tau.true = -0.3, prob.cens = 35%, $V \sim Unif(0, \sqrt{12})$, size = 500

	$\hat{\bar{\beta}}_V$	$med(\hat{\beta}_V)$	$sd(\hat{\beta}_V)$	$\overline{sd(\hat{\beta}_V)}$	$\% \in$ CI	$\widehat{MSE}$	$\widehat{\mathbb{E}(T)}$
sd.U = 0							
benchmark	-0.201	-0.202	0.042	0.042	95.000	0.002	0.649
naive	-0.201	-0.202	0.042	0.042	95.000	0.002	0.649
reg.calib	-0.201	-0.202	0.042	0.042	95.000	0.002	0.649
corr	-0.201	-0.202	0.042	0.042	94.600	0.002	0.649
sd.U = 0.1							
benchmark	-0.202	-0.201	0.042	0.042	95.300	0.002	0.648
naive	-0.200	-0.199	0.041	0.041	95.700	0.002	0.650
reg.calib	-0.202	-0.201	0.042	0.042	95.600	0.002	0.648
corr	-0.202	-0.201	0.042	0.042	95.200	0.002	0.648
sd.U = 0.4							
benchmark	-0.201	-0.200	0.041	0.042	96.000	0.002	0.649
naive	-0.174	-0.173	0.038	0.039	88.900	0.002	0.681
reg.calib	-0.201	-0.201	0.044	0.045	96.000	0.002	0.649
corr	-0.202	-0.200	0.045	0.045	95.900	0.002	0.649
sd.U = 0.8							
benchmark	-0.202	-0.200	0.042	0.042	94.800	0.002	0.648
naive	-0.124	-0.125	0.033	0.033	35.600	0.007	0.742
reg.calib	-0.205	-0.205	0.055	0.054	93.100	0.003	0.647
corr	-0.206	-0.207	0.057	0.056	93.800	0.003	0.645

	$\hat{\bar{\tau}}$	$med(\hat{\tau})$	$sd(\hat{\tau})$	$\overline{sd(\hat{\tau})}$	$\% \in$ CI	$\widehat{MSE}$	#NA
sd.U = 0							
benchmark	-0.302	-0.301	0.044	0.044	94.900	0.002	0
naive	-0.302	-0.301	0.044	0.044	94.900	0.002	0
reg.calib	-0.302	-0.301	0.044	0.044	94.900	0.002	0
corr	-0.302	-0.301	0.044	0.044	94.900	0.002	0
sd.U = 0.1							
benchmark	-0.303	-0.303	0.044	0.044	95.100	0.002	0
naive	-0.303	-0.302	0.044	0.044	95.100	0.002	0
reg.calib	-0.303	-0.302	0.044	0.044	95.100	0.002	0
corr	-0.303	-0.303	0.044	0.044	95.300	0.002	0
sd.U = 0.4							
benchmark	-0.304	-0.305	0.044	0.044	94.600	0.002	0
naive	-0.301	-0.300	0.044	0.044	94.500	0.002	0
reg.calib	-0.301	-0.300	0.044	0.044	94.500	0.002	0
corr	-0.305	-0.304	0.045	0.044	94.600	0.002	0
sd.U = 0.8							
benchmark	-0.305	-0.306	0.041	0.044	96.600	0.002	0
naive	-0.295	-0.293	0.041	0.044	96.500	0.002	0
reg.calib	-0.295	-0.293	0.041	0.044	96.500	0.002	0
corr	-0.307	-0.307	0.043	0.045	96.300	0.002	0

Table C.5.: Results for β_V and τ with `beta.true` = -0.2, `tau.true` = -0.3, `prob.cens` = 35%, $V \sim Unif(0, \sqrt{12})$ and `size` = 500

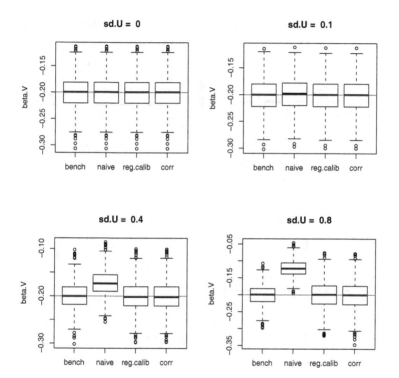

Figure C.11.: Boxplot for β_V with beta.true = -0.2, tau.true = -0.3, prob.cens = 35%, $V \sim Unif(0, \sqrt{12})$, size = 1000

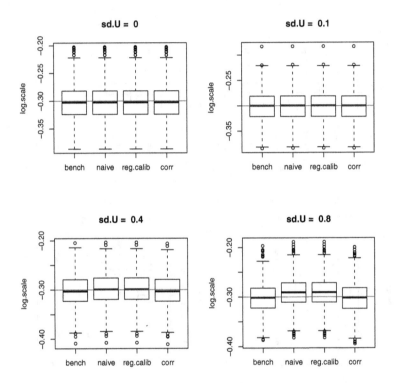

Figure C.12.: Boxplot for τ with beta.true = -0.2, tau.true = -0.3, prob.cens = 35%, $V \sim Unif(0, \sqrt{12})$, size = 1000

	$\tilde{\hat{\beta}}_V$	$med(\hat{\beta}_V)$	$sd(\hat{\beta}_V)$	$\overline{sd(\hat{\beta}_V)}$	$\% \in$ CI	$\widehat{MSE}$	$\widehat{E(T)}$
sd.U $= 0$							
benchmark	-0.200	-0.199	0.030	0.029	94.700	0.001	0.649
naive	-0.200	-0.199	0.030	0.029	94.700	0.001	0.649
reg.calib	-0.200	-0.199	0.030	0.029	94.700	0.001	0.649
corr	-0.200	-0.199	0.030	0.029	94.400	0.001	0.649
sd.U $= 0.1$							
benchmark	-0.201	-0.200	0.029	0.029	94.900	0.001	0.649
naive	-0.199	-0.198	0.029	0.029	95.300	0.001	0.651
reg.calib	-0.201	-0.200	0.030	0.030	95.100	0.001	0.649
corr	-0.201	-0.200	0.030	0.030	95.000	0.001	0.649
sd.U $= 0.4$							
benchmark	-0.200	-0.200	0.029	0.029	96.000	0.001	0.650
naive	-0.172	-0.173	0.027	0.027	82.800	0.001	0.681
reg.calib	-0.200	-0.202	0.031	0.032	95.200	0.001	0.650
corr	-0.200	-0.202	0.031	0.032	95.100	0.001	0.649
sd.U $= 0.8$							
benchmark	-0.201	-0.199	0.029	0.029	94.300	0.001	0.648
naive	-0.122	-0.122	0.023	0.023	8.700	0.007	0.744
reg.calib	-0.201	-0.199	0.039	0.038	95.000	0.002	0.650
corr	-0.202	-0.200	0.040	0.039	95.500	0.002	0.648

	$\tilde{\hat{\tau}}$	$med(\hat{\tau})$	$sd(\hat{\tau})$	$\overline{sd(\hat{\tau})}$	$\% \in$ CI	$\widehat{MSE}$	#NA
sd.U $= 0$							
benchmark	-0.302	-0.303	0.031	0.031	93.900	0.001	0
naive	-0.302	-0.303	0.031	0.031	93.900	0.001	0
reg.calib	-0.302	-0.303	0.031	0.031	93.900	0.001	0
corr	-0.302	-0.303	0.031	0.031	94.300	0.001	0
sd.U $= 0.1$							
benchmark	-0.301	-0.300	0.030	0.031	96.100	0.001	0
naive	-0.300	-0.300	0.030	0.031	95.900	0.001	0
reg.calib	-0.300	-0.300	0.030	0.031	95.900	0.001	0
corr	-0.301	-0.300	0.030	0.031	96.100	0.001	0
sd.U $= 0.4$							
benchmark	-0.301	-0.303	0.031	0.031	95.700	0.001	0
naive	-0.298	-0.299	0.031	0.031	95.300	0.001	0
reg.calib	-0.298	-0.299	0.031	0.031	95.300	0.001	0
corr	-0.302	-0.303	0.032	0.031	95.200	0.001	0
sd.U $= 0.8$							
benchmark	-0.301	-0.301	0.030	0.031	94.500	0.001	0
naive	-0.291	-0.291	0.031	0.031	94.100	0.001	0
reg.calib	-0.291	-0.291	0.031	0.031	94.100	0.001	0
corr	-0.302	-0.302	0.031	0.032	94.800	0.001	0

Table C.6.: Results for β_V and τ with beta.true = -0.2, tau.true = -0.3, prob.cens = 35%, $V \sim Unif(0, \sqrt{12})$ and size = 1000

C.1.3. beta.true = 0.4, tau.true = 0.5, prob.cens = 0% and $V \sim N(0,1)$

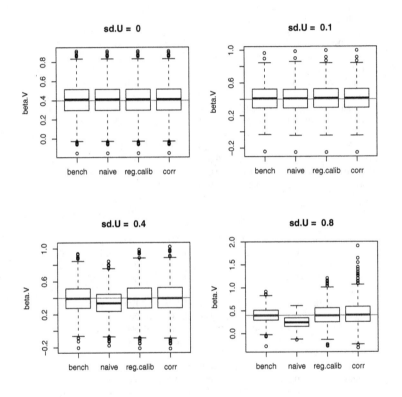

Figure C.13.: Boxplot for β_V with beta.true = 0.4, tau.true = 0.5, prob.cens = 0%, $V \sim N(0,1)$, size = 100

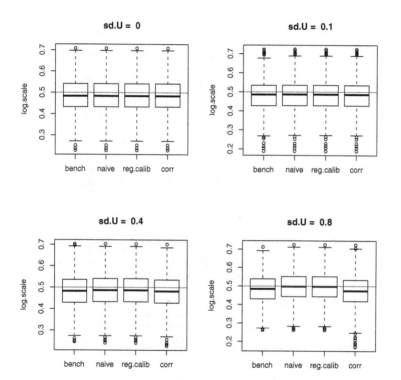

Figure C.14.: Boxplot for τ with beta.true $= 0.4$, tau.true $= 0.5$ prob.cens $= 0\%$,
        $V \sim N(0, 1)$, size $= 100$

	$\hat{\bar{\beta}}_V$	$med(\hat{\beta}_V)$	$sd(\hat{\beta}_V)$	$\overline{sd(\hat{\beta}_V)}$	$\% \in$ CI	$\widehat{MSE}$	$\widehat{\mathbb{E}(T)}$
sd.U $= 0$							
benchmark	0.407	0.412	0.165	0.166	95.600	0.027	1.478
naive	0.407	0.412	0.165	0.166	95.600	0.027	1.478
reg.calib	0.407	0.412	0.165	0.166	95.600	0.027	1.478
corr	0.407	0.412	0.165	0.158	93.400	0.027	1.478
sd.U $= 0.1$							
benchmark	0.406	0.411	0.172	0.166	94.000	0.029	1.471
naive	0.401	0.409	0.171	0.165	93.600	0.029	1.472
reg.calib	0.405	0.413	0.173	0.167	93.900	0.030	1.472
corr	0.405	0.413	0.173	0.159	90.600	0.030	1.471
sd.U $= 0.4$							
benchmark	0.392	0.395	0.171	0.167	94.200	0.029	1.469
naive	0.339	0.337	0.159	0.156	92.400	0.029	1.477
reg.calib	0.395	0.394	0.187	0.182	94.300	0.035	1.478
corr	0.398	0.397	0.189	0.175	92.800	0.036	1.467
sd.U $= 0.8$							
benchmark	0.400	0.399	0.161	0.167	95.900	0.026	1.474
naive	0.245	0.243	0.134	0.132	76.700	0.042	1.496
reg.calib	0.409	0.395	0.233	0.222	93.800	0.055	1.499
corr	0.433	0.406	0.267	0.238	94.394	0.072	1.460

	$\hat{\bar{\tau}}$	$med(\hat{\tau})$	$sd(\hat{\tau})$	$\overline{sd(\hat{\tau})}$	$\% \in$ CI	$\widehat{MSE}$	#NA
sd.U $= 0$							
benchmark	0.485	0.484	0.079	0.078	95.200	0.006	0
naive	0.485	0.484	0.079	0.078	95.200	0.006	0
reg.calib	0.485	0.484	0.079	0.078	95.200	0.006	0
corr	0.485	0.484	0.079	0.076	94.600	0.006	0
sd.U $= 0.1$							
benchmark	0.482	0.486	0.082	0.078	92.900	0.007	0
naive	0.482	0.487	0.082	0.078	93.500	0.007	0
reg.calib	0.482	0.487	0.082	0.078	93.500	0.007	0
corr	0.482	0.486	0.082	0.077	91.900	0.007	0
sd.U $= 0.4$							
benchmark	0.482	0.483	0.079	0.078	92.800	0.007	0
naive	0.486	0.486	0.079	0.078	94.100	0.006	0
reg.calib	0.486	0.486	0.079	0.078	94.100	0.006	0
corr	0.480	0.482	0.080	0.077	92.300	0.007	0
sd.U $= 0.8$							
benchmark	0.483	0.484	0.078	0.078	93.900	0.006	0
naive	0.496	0.498	0.079	0.078	94.000	0.006	0
reg.calib	0.496	0.498	0.079	0.078	94.000	0.006	0
corr	0.473	0.474	0.086	0.084	92.492	0.008	1

Table C.7.: Results for β_V and τ with beta.true $= 0.4$, tau.true $= 0.5$, prob.cens $=$ 0%, $V \sim N(0,1)$ and size $= 100$

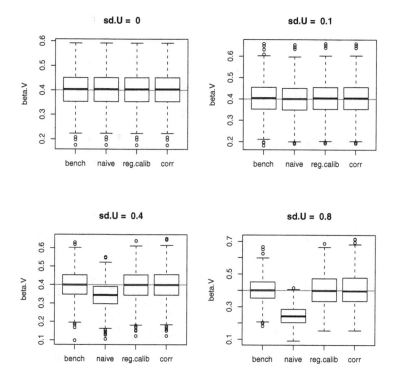

Figure C.15.: Boxplot for β_V with beta.true $= 0.4$, tau.true $= 0.5$, prob.cens $= 0\%$, $V \sim N(0,1)$, size $= 500$

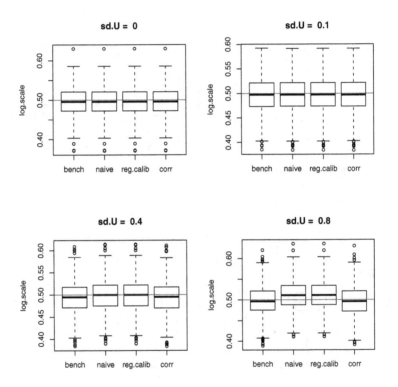

Figure C.16.: Boxplot for τ with beta.true = 0.4, tau.true = 0.5, prob.cens = 0%, $V \sim N(0,1)$, size = 500

	$\bar{\hat{\beta}}_V$	$med(\hat{\beta}_V)$	$sd(\hat{\beta}_V)$	$\overline{sd}(\hat{\beta}_V)$	$\% \in$ CI	$\widehat{MSE}$	$\widehat{\mathbb{E}(T)}$
sd.U $= 0$							
benchmark	0.401	0.404	0.071	0.074	96.000	0.005	1.481
naive	0.401	0.404	0.071	0.074	96.000	0.005	1.481
reg.calib	0.401	0.404	0.071	0.074	96.000	0.005	1.481
corr	0.401	0.404	0.071	0.073	95.300	0.005	1.481
sd.U $= 0.1$							
benchmark	0.403	0.404	0.075	0.074	94.200	0.006	1.483
naive	0.399	0.401	0.075	0.074	94.300	0.006	1.484
reg.calib	0.403	0.405	0.076	0.074	94.500	0.006	1.484
corr	0.403	0.404	0.076	0.074	93.500	0.006	1.483
sd.U $= 0.4$							
benchmark	0.400	0.400	0.078	0.074	93.300	0.006	1.478
naive	0.344	0.344	0.072	0.069	86.500	0.008	1.487
reg.calib	0.399	0.400	0.083	0.080	93.600	0.007	1.487
corr	0.399	0.400	0.083	0.079	93.600	0.007	1.478
sd.U $= 0.8$							
benchmark	0.401	0.400	0.073	0.074	94.600	0.005	1.485
naive	0.244	0.243	0.059	0.059	25.600	0.028	1.512
reg.calib	0.401	0.398	0.099	0.097	94.500	0.010	1.512
corr	0.405	0.397	0.103	0.100	94.400	0.011	1.483

	$\bar{\hat{\tau}}$	$med(\hat{\tau})$	$sd(\hat{\tau})$	$\overline{sd}(\hat{\tau})$	$\% \in$ CI	$\widehat{MSE}$	#NA
sd.U $= 0$							
benchmark	0.496	0.496	0.036	0.035	94.500	0.001	0
naive	0.496	0.496	0.036	0.035	94.500	0.001	0
reg.calib	0.496	0.496	0.036	0.035	94.500	0.001	0
corr	0.496	0.496	0.036	0.035	94.500	0.001	0
sd.U $= 0.1$							
benchmark	0.497	0.497	0.035	0.035	94.200	0.001	0
naive	0.498	0.498	0.035	0.035	94.500	0.001	0
reg.calib	0.498	0.498	0.035	0.035	94.500	0.001	0
corr	0.497	0.497	0.035	0.035	94.400	0.001	0
sd.U $= 0.4$							
benchmark	0.495	0.495	0.036	0.035	94.100	0.001	0
naive	0.500	0.500	0.036	0.035	93.800	0.001	0
reg.calib	0.500	0.500	0.036	0.035	93.800	0.001	0
corr	0.495	0.495	0.036	0.035	93.600	0.001	0
sd.U $= 0.8$							
benchmark	0.498	0.497	0.035	0.035	94.600	0.001	0
naive	0.512	0.511	0.035	0.035	92.700	0.001	0
reg.calib	0.512	0.511	0.035	0.035	92.700	0.001	0
corr	0.497	0.496	0.037	0.036	94.500	0.001	0

Table C.8.: Results for β_V and τ with `beta.true` $= 0.4$, `tau.true` $= 0.5$, `prob.cens` $= 0\%$, $V \sim N(0,1)$ and `size` $= 500$

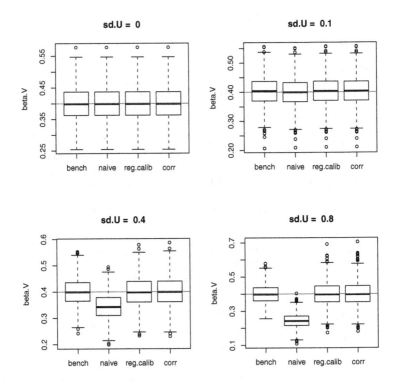

Figure C.17.: Boxplot for β_V with beta.true $= 0.4$, tau.true $= 0.5$, prob.cens $= 0\%$, $V \sim N(0,1)$, size $= 1000$

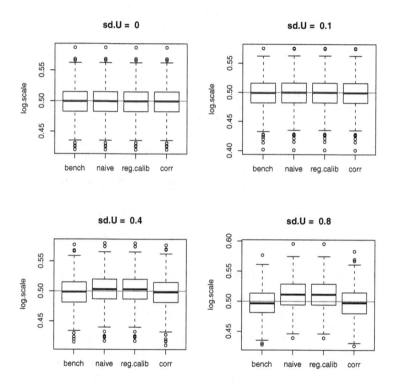

Figure C.18.: Boxplot for τ with beta.true $= 0.4$, tau.true $= 0.5$, prob.cens $= 0\%$, $V \sim N(0,1)$, size $= 1000$

	$\hat{\bar{\beta}}_V$	$med(\hat{\beta}_V)$	$sd(\hat{\beta}_V)$	$\overline{sd(\hat{\beta}_V)}$	% $\in$ CI	$\widehat{MSE}$	$\widehat{\mathbb{E}(T)}$
sd.U $= 0$							
benchmark	0.400	0.399	0.053	0.052	94.500	0.003	1.483
naive	0.400	0.399	0.053	0.052	94.500	0.003	1.483
reg.calib	0.400	0.399	0.053	0.052	94.500	0.003	1.483
corr	0.400	0.399	0.053	0.052	94.300	0.003	1.483
sd.U $= 0.1$							
benchmark	0.404	0.404	0.051	0.052	95.700	0.003	1.483
naive	0.400	0.400	0.050	0.052	95.300	0.003	1.484
reg.calib	0.404	0.404	0.051	0.052	95.500	0.003	1.484
corr	0.404	0.403	0.051	0.052	95.300	0.003	1.483
sd.U $= 0.4$							
benchmark	0.399	0.399	0.052	0.052	95.300	0.003	1.482
naive	0.344	0.343	0.048	0.049	79.000	0.005	1.492
reg.calib	0.400	0.398	0.056	0.057	95.400	0.003	1.492
corr	0.400	0.399	0.056	0.057	95.600	0.003	1.482
sd.U $= 0.8$							
benchmark	0.399	0.398	0.055	0.052	94.000	0.003	1.481
naive	0.242	0.242	0.043	0.041	3.800	0.027	1.508
reg.calib	0.399	0.397	0.072	0.068	94.300	0.005	1.508
corr	0.401	0.397	0.074	0.070	93.400	0.005	1.480

	$\hat{\bar{\tau}}$	$med(\hat{\tau})$	$sd(\hat{\tau})$	$\overline{sd(\hat{\tau})}$	% $\in$ CI	$\widehat{MSE}$	#NA
sd.U $= 0$							
benchmark	0.499	0.500	0.025	0.025	95.200	0.001	0
naive	0.499	0.500	0.025	0.025	95.200	0.001	0
reg.calib	0.499	0.500	0.025	0.025	95.200	0.001	0
corr	0.499	0.500	0.025	0.025	95.100	0.001	0
sd.U $= 0.1$							
benchmark	0.499	0.499	0.025	0.025	94.900	0.001	0
naive	0.499	0.500	0.025	0.025	95.000	0.001	0
reg.calib	0.499	0.500	0.025	0.025	95.000	0.001	0
corr	0.499	0.499	0.025	0.025	94.900	0.001	0
sd.U $= 0.4$							
benchmark	0.498	0.499	0.024	0.025	95.100	0.001	0
naive	0.503	0.503	0.025	0.025	94.800	0.001	0
reg.calib	0.503	0.503	0.025	0.025	94.800	0.001	0
corr	0.498	0.498	0.025	0.025	95.100	0.001	0
sd.U $= 0.8$							
benchmark	0.498	0.497	0.024	0.025	96.100	0.001	0
naive	0.511	0.511	0.024	0.025	93.400	0.001	0
reg.calib	0.511	0.511	0.024	0.025	93.400	0.001	0
corr	0.497	0.497	0.025	0.026	96.000	0.001	0

Table C.9.: Results for β_V and τ with `beta.true` $= 0.4$, `tau.true` $= 0.5$, `prob.cens` $=$ 0%, $V \sim N(0,1)$ and `size` $= 1000$

C.1.4. beta.true $= 0.4$, tau.true $= 0.5$, prob.cens $= 0\%$ and $V \sim Unif(0, \sqrt{12})$

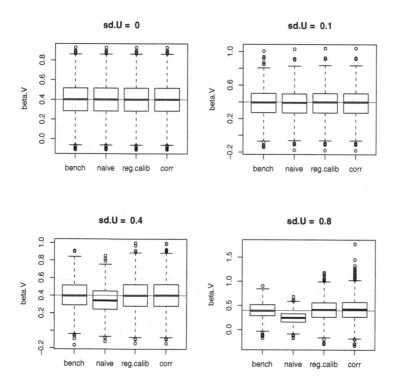

Figure C.19.: Boxplot for β_V with beta.true $= 0.4$, tau.true $= 0.5$, prob.cens $= 0\%$, $V \sim Unif(0, \sqrt{12})$, size $= 100$

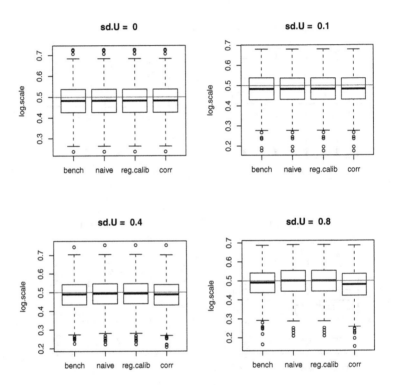

Figure C.20.: Boxplot for τ with beta.true $= 0.4$, tau.true $= 0.5$, prob.cens $= 0\%$, $V \sim Unif(0, \sqrt{12})$, size $= 100$

	$\bar{\hat{\beta}}_V$	$med(\hat{\beta}_V)$	$sd(\hat{\beta}_V)$	$\overline{sd}(\hat{\beta}_V)$	$\% \in$ CI	$\widehat{MSE}$	$\widehat{\mathbb{E}(T)}$
sd.U = 0							
benchmark	0.401	0.402	0.172	0.165	93.600	0.029	3.067
naive	0.401	0.402	0.172	0.165	93.600	0.029	3.067
reg.calib	0.401	0.402	0.172	0.165	93.600	0.029	3.067
corr	0.401	0.402	0.172	0.159	92.300	0.029	3.067
sd.U = 0.1							
benchmark	0.388	0.396	0.168	0.164	94.300	0.028	3.002
naive	0.384	0.394	0.167	0.164	94.500	0.028	2.981
reg.calib	0.387	0.398	0.168	0.165	94.500	0.028	3.003
corr	0.388	0.398	0.168	0.161	93.300	0.028	3.002
sd.U = 0.4							
benchmark	0.402	0.397	0.168	0.166	93.900	0.028	3.091
naive	0.345	0.343	0.159	0.155	92.700	0.028	2.810
reg.calib	0.401	0.400	0.186	0.180	93.300	0.034	3.141
corr	0.403	0.400	0.188	0.175	92.400	0.035	3.124
sd.U = 0.8							
benchmark	0.398	0.393	0.164	0.166	94.900	0.027	3.065
naive	0.249	0.250	0.130	0.133	79.000	0.040	2.369
reg.calib	0.417	0.413	0.225	0.223	94.800	0.051	3.337
corr	0.433	0.425	0.245	0.236	94.885	0.061	3.378

	$\bar{\hat{\tau}}$	$med(\hat{\tau})$	$sd(\hat{\tau})$	$\overline{sd}(\hat{\tau})$	$\% \in$ CI	$\widehat{MSE}$	#NA
sd.U = 0							
benchmark	0.481	0.483	0.081	0.078	93.900	0.007	0
naive	0.481	0.483	0.081	0.078	93.900	0.007	0
reg.calib	0.481	0.483	0.081	0.078	93.900	0.007	0
corr	0.481	0.483	0.081	0.076	92.400	0.007	0
sd.U = 0.1							
benchmark	0.482	0.483	0.078	0.078	94.000	0.006	0
naive	0.482	0.483	0.078	0.078	94.400	0.006	0
reg.calib	0.482	0.483	0.078	0.078	94.400	0.006	0
corr	0.481	0.483	0.078	0.076	93.900	0.006	0
sd.U = 0.4							
benchmark	0.488	0.491	0.080	0.078	94.300	0.007	0
naive	0.493	0.494	0.080	0.078	94.100	0.006	0
reg.calib	0.493	0.494	0.080	0.078	94.100	0.006	0
corr	0.486	0.488	0.081	0.077	93.200	0.007	0
sd.U = 0.8							
benchmark	0.487	0.491	0.078	0.078	94.900	0.006	0
naive	0.499	0.501	0.077	0.078	95.500	0.006	0
reg.calib	0.499	0.501	0.077	0.078	95.500	0.006	0
corr	0.478	0.481	0.083	0.083	94.784	0.007	3

Table C.10.: Results for β_V and τ with `beta.true` = 0.4, `tau.true` = 0.5, `prob.cens` = 0%, $V \sim Unif(0, \sqrt{12})$ and `size` = 100

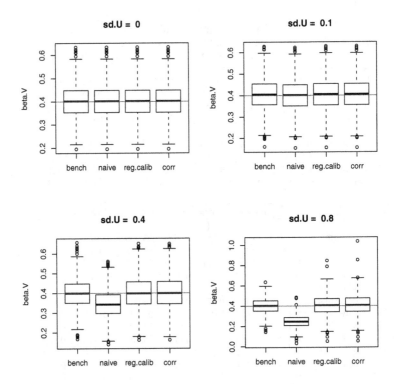

Figure C.21.: Boxplot for β_V with `beta.true` $= 0.4$, `tau.true` $= 0.5$, `prob.cens` $= 0\%$, $V \sim Unif(0, \sqrt{12})$, `size` $= 500$

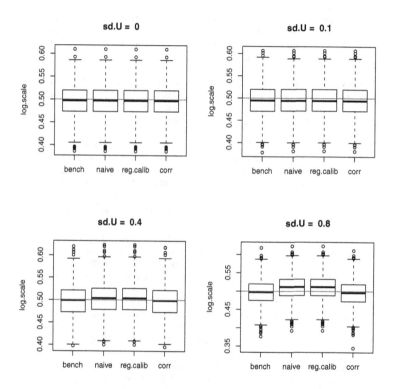

Figure C.22.: Boxplot for τ with beta.true $= 0.4$, tau.true $= 0.5$, prob.cens $= 0\%$, $V \sim Unif(0, \sqrt{12})$, size $= 500$

	$\hat{\bar{\beta}}_V$	$med(\hat{\beta}_V)$	$sd(\hat{\beta}_V)$	$\overline{sd(\hat{\beta}_V)}$	$\% \in$ CI	$\widehat{MSE}$	$\widehat{\mathbb{E}(T)}$
sd.U $= 0$							
benchmark	0.401	0.401	0.073	0.074	95.000	0.005	2.987
naive	0.401	0.401	0.073	0.074	95.000	0.005	2.987
reg.calib	0.401	0.401	0.073	0.074	95.000	0.005	2.987
corr	0.401	0.401	0.073	0.073	94.400	0.005	2.987
sd.U $= 0.1$							
benchmark	0.404	0.405	0.074	0.073	94.500	0.005	3.006
naive	0.400	0.402	0.074	0.073	94.100	0.005	2.988
reg.calib	0.404	0.406	0.074	0.074	94.100	0.006	3.009
corr	0.404	0.406	0.074	0.074	94.000	0.006	3.008
sd.U $= 0.4$							
benchmark	0.401	0.400	0.073	0.074	95.400	0.005	2.994
naive	0.345	0.343	0.068	0.069	88.200	0.008	2.734
reg.calib	0.400	0.399	0.080	0.080	94.700	0.006	3.017
corr	0.401	0.399	0.080	0.080	94.900	0.006	2.998
sd.U $= 0.8$							
benchmark	0.400	0.402	0.074	0.074	94.700	0.005	2.989
naive	0.246	0.245	0.059	0.059	25.100	0.027	2.320
reg.calib	0.404	0.405	0.097	0.096	95.000	0.009	3.082
corr	0.407	0.405	0.102	0.100	95.600	0.010	3.042

	$\hat{\bar{\tau}}$	$med(\hat{\tau})$	$sd(\hat{\tau})$	$\overline{sd(\hat{\tau})}$	$\% \in$ CI	$\widehat{MSE}$	#NA
sd.U $= 0$							
benchmark	0.497	0.497	0.034	0.035	95.900	0.001	0
naive	0.497	0.497	0.034	0.035	95.900	0.001	0
reg.calib	0.497	0.497	0.034	0.035	95.900	0.001	0
corr	0.497	0.497	0.034	0.035	95.400	0.001	0
sd.U $= 0.1$							
benchmark	0.495	0.495	0.036	0.035	92.800	0.001	0
naive	0.495	0.495	0.036	0.035	92.700	0.001	0
reg.calib	0.495	0.495	0.036	0.035	92.700	0.001	0
corr	0.495	0.494	0.037	0.035	92.700	0.001	0
sd.U $= 0.4$							
benchmark	0.498	0.499	0.035	0.035	94.900	0.001	0
naive	0.503	0.504	0.035	0.035	94.600	0.001	0
reg.calib	0.503	0.504	0.035	0.035	94.600	0.001	0
corr	0.498	0.499	0.036	0.035	95.000	0.001	0
sd.U $= 0.8$							
benchmark	0.497	0.498	0.034	0.035	95.800	0.001	0
naive	0.511	0.512	0.034	0.035	95.100	0.001	0
reg.calib	0.511	0.512	0.034	0.035	95.100	0.001	0
corr	0.495	0.496	0.036	0.037	95.100	0.001	0

Table C.11.: Results for β_V and τ with beta.true $= 0.4$, tau.true $= 0.5$, prob.cens $= 0\%$, $V \sim Unif(0, \sqrt{12})$ and size $= 500$

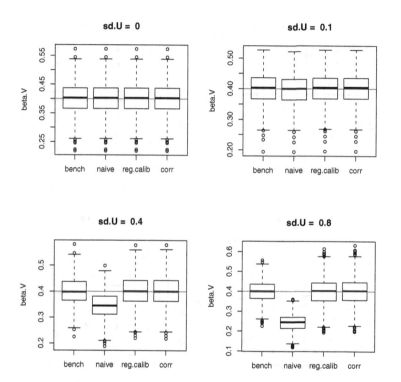

Figure C.23.: Boxplot for β_V with beta.true $= 0.4$, tau.true $= 0.5$, prob.cens $= 0\%$, $V \sim Unif(0, \sqrt{12})$, size $= 1000$

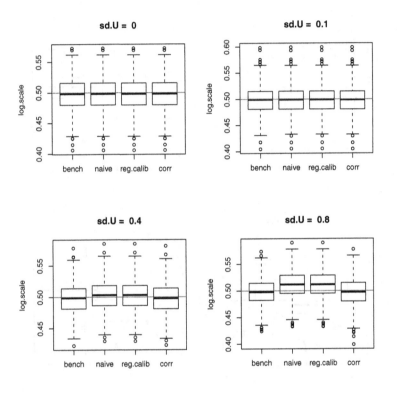

Figure C.24.: Boxplot for τ with beta.true $= 0.4$, tau.true $= 0.5$, prob.cens $= 0\%$, $V \sim Unif(0, \sqrt{12})$, size $= 1000$

	$\tilde{\bar{\beta}}_V$	$med(\hat{\beta}_V)$	$sd(\hat{\beta}_V)$	$\overline{sd(\hat{\beta}_V)}$	$\% \in$ CI	$\widehat{MSE}$	$\widehat{E(T)}$
sd.U $= 0$							
benchmark	0.402	0.403	0.052	0.052	95.300	0.003	2.982
naive	0.402	0.403	0.052	0.052	95.300	0.003	2.982
reg.calib	0.402	0.403	0.052	0.052	95.300	0.003	2.982
corr	0.402	0.403	0.052	0.052	95.400	0.003	2.982
sd.U $= 0.1$							
benchmark	0.402	0.404	0.051	0.052	95.800	0.003	2.985
naive	0.397	0.400	0.051	0.052	95.400	0.003	2.964
reg.calib	0.401	0.404	0.052	0.052	95.000	0.003	2.984
corr	0.401	0.404	0.052	0.052	94.900	0.003	2.983
sd.U $= 0.4$							
benchmark	0.400	0.398	0.052	0.052	95.100	0.003	2.975
naive	0.346	0.345	0.048	0.049	79.900	0.005	2.722
reg.calib	0.401	0.401	0.056	0.056	96.200	0.003	3.000
corr	0.402	0.400	0.056	0.056	96.400	0.003	2.981
sd.U $= 0.8$							
benchmark	0.400	0.401	0.051	0.052	94.800	0.003	2.977
naive	0.244	0.246	0.041	0.041	4.000	0.026	2.310
reg.calib	0.402	0.403	0.068	0.068	94.700	0.005	3.049
corr	0.403	0.403	0.069	0.070	95.300	0.005	2.999

	$\tilde{\bar{\tau}}$	$med(\hat{\tau})$	$sd(\hat{\tau})$	$\overline{sd(\hat{\tau})}$	$\% \in$ CI	$\widehat{MSE}$	#NA
sd.U $= 0$							
benchmark	0.498	0.498	0.025	0.025	95.500	0.001	0
naive	0.498	0.498	0.025	0.025	95.500	0.001	0
reg.calib	0.498	0.498	0.025	0.025	95.500	0.001	0
corr	0.498	0.498	0.025	0.025	94.800	0.001	0
sd.U $= 0.1$							
benchmark	0.498	0.499	0.025	0.025	94.600	0.001	0
naive	0.499	0.499	0.025	0.025	94.600	0.001	0
reg.calib	0.499	0.499	0.025	0.025	94.600	0.001	0
corr	0.498	0.499	0.025	0.025	94.200	0.001	0
sd.U $= 0.4$							
benchmark	0.498	0.499	0.024	0.025	94.600	0.001	0
naive	0.503	0.503	0.024	0.025	94.500	0.001	0
reg.calib	0.503	0.503	0.024	0.025	94.500	0.001	0
corr	0.498	0.498	0.025	0.025	95.100	0.001	0
sd.U $= 0.8$							
benchmark	0.498	0.498	0.024	0.025	95.100	0.001	0
naive	0.512	0.512	0.024	0.025	93.100	0.001	0
reg.calib	0.512	0.512	0.024	0.025	93.100	0.001	0
corr	0.497	0.497	0.026	0.026	95.200	0.001	0

Table C.12.: Results for β_V and τ with `beta.true` $= 0.4$, `tau.true` $= 0.5$, `prob.cens` $= 0\%$, $V \sim Unif(0, \sqrt{12})$ and `size` $= 1000$

C.2. Check the `fit` function - W and F

C.2.1. `beta.V.true` = **0.6**, `beta.F.true` = **-0.1**, `tau.true` = **-0.5**, `prob.cens` = **0%** and $V \sim N(0,1)$

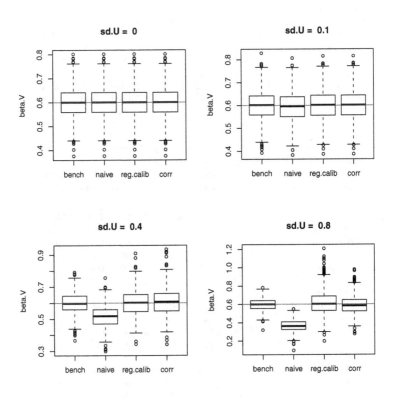

Figure C.25.: Boxplot for β_V with `beta.V.true` = 0.6, `beta.F.true` = -0.1, `tau.true` = -0.5, `prob.cens` = 0%, $V \sim N(0,1)$, `size` = 100

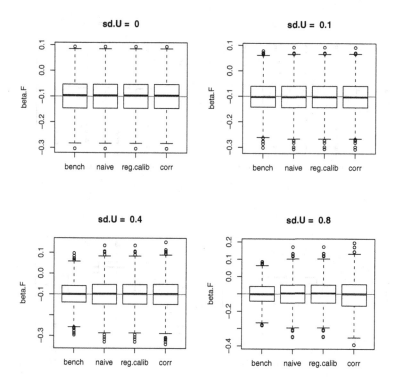

Figure C.26.: Boxplot for β_F with beta.V.true $= 0.6$, beta.F.true $= -0.1$, tau.true $= -0.5$, prob.cens $= 0\%$, $V \sim N(0,1)$, size $= 100$

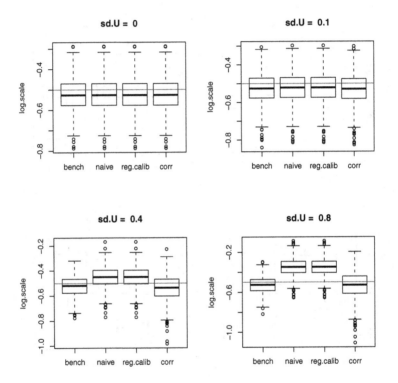

Figure C.27.: Boxplot for τ with beta.V.true = 0.6, beta.F.true = -0.1, tau.true = -0.5, prob.cens = 0%, $V \sim N(0,1)$, size = 100

	$\hat{\beta}_V$	$med(\hat{\beta}_V)$	$sd(\hat{\beta}_V)$	$sd(\hat{\beta}_V)$	$\% \in CI$	$\widehat{MSE}$	$\hat{\beta}_F$	$med(\hat{\beta}_F)$	$sd(\hat{\beta}_F)$	$sd(\hat{\beta}_F)$	$\% \in CI$	$\widehat{MSE}$	$\widehat{\mathbb{E}(T)}$
sd.U = 0													
benchmark	0.600	0.600	0.062	0.061	94.400	0.004	-0.098	-0.097	0.064	0.062	93.900	0.004	0.896
naive	0.600	0.600	0.062	0.061	94.400	0.004	-0.098	-0.097	0.064	0.062	93.900	0.004	0.896
reg.calib	0.600	0.600	0.062	0.061	94.400	0.004	-0.098	-0.097	0.064	0.062	93.900	0.004	0.896
corr	0.600	0.600	0.062	0.058	92.100	0.004	-0.098	-0.097	0.064	0.058	92.400	0.004	0.896
sd.U = 0.1													
benchmark	0.599	0.602	0.063	0.061	94.000	0.004	-0.101	-0.102	0.063	0.061	93.500	0.004	0.897
naive	0.593	0.596	0.063	0.061	93.800	0.004	-0.102	-0.102	0.063	0.061	93.200	0.004	0.897
reg.calib	0.600	0.602	0.064	0.062	94.400	0.004	-0.102	-0.102	0.063	0.061	93.200	0.004	0.897
corr	0.600	0.602	0.064	0.058	92.500	0.004	-0.102	-0.102	0.063	0.058	91.500	0.004	0.897
sd.U = 0.4													
benchmark	0.599	0.597	0.063	0.062	94.400	0.004	-0.100	-0.100	0.061	0.061	95.000	0.004	0.895
naive	0.516	0.519	0.065	0.061	69.600	0.011	-0.099	-0.098	0.069	0.066	93.900	0.005	0.900
reg.calib	0.601	0.602	0.077	0.071	94.100	0.006	-0.099	-0.098	0.069	0.066	93.900	0.005	0.900
corr	0.608	0.607	0.081	0.072	92.000	0.007	-0.098	-0.098	0.071	0.065	92.900	0.005	0.894
sd.U = 0.8													
benchmark	0.598	0.600	0.062	0.061	94.400	0.004	-0.100	-0.101	0.062	0.061	94.200	0.004	0.898
naive	0.366	0.363	0.063	0.057	3.200	0.059	-0.099	-0.096	0.078	0.073	93.200	0.006	0.914
reg.calib	0.615	0.603	0.126	0.097	87.600	0.016	-0.099	-0.096	0.078	0.073	93.200	0.006	0.917
corr	0.585	0.584	0.100	0.144	94.828	0.010	-0.103	-0.100	0.096	0.088	92.006	0.009	0.898

Table C.13.: Results for β_V and β_F with beta.V.true = 0.6, beta.F.true = -0.1, tau.true = -0.5, prob.cens = 0%, $V \sim N(0,1)$ and size = 100

	$\bar{\hat{\tau}}$	$med(\hat{\tau})$	$sd(\hat{\tau})$	$\overline{sd(\hat{\tau})}$	$\% \in$ CI	$\widehat{MSE}$	#NA
sd.U $= 0$							
benchmark	-0.525	-0.526	0.078	0.078	94.000	0.007	0
naive	-0.525	-0.526	0.078	0.078	94.000	0.007	0
reg.calib	-0.525	-0.526	0.078	0.078	94.000	0.007	0
corr	-0.525	-0.526	0.078	0.077	93.200	0.007	0
sd.U $= 0.1$							
benchmark	-0.527	-0.526	0.079	0.079	94.200	0.007	0
naive	-0.521	-0.522	0.079	0.078	93.800	0.007	0
reg.calib	-0.521	-0.522	0.079	0.078	93.800	0.007	0
corr	-0.528	-0.530	0.080	0.077	92.400	0.007	0
sd.U $= 0.4$							
benchmark	-0.522	-0.519	0.080	0.078	93.300	0.007	0
naive	-0.452	-0.450	0.081	0.078	89.200	0.009	0
reg.calib	-0.452	-0.450	0.081	0.078	89.200	0.009	0
corr	-0.540	-0.537	0.102	0.093	92.400	0.012	0
sd.U $= 0.8$							
benchmark	-0.527	-0.526	0.079	0.078	93.800	0.007	0
naive	-0.350	-0.349	0.083	0.076	49.500	0.029	0
reg.calib	-0.350	-0.349	0.083	0.076	49.500	0.029	0
corr	-0.539	-0.529	0.136	0.180	98.119	0.020	362

Table C.14.: Results for τ with beta.V.true $= 0.6$, beta.F.true $= -0.1$, tau.true $=$ -0.5, prob.cens $= 0\%$, $V \sim N(0,1)$ and size $= 100$

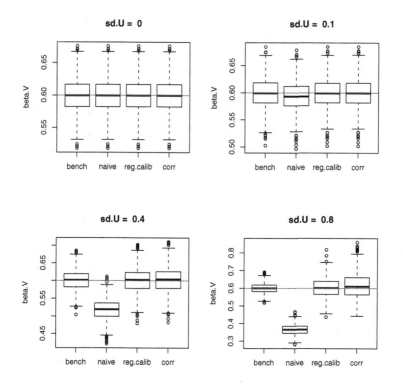

Figure C.28.: Boxplot for β_V with beta.V.true $= 0.6$, beta.F.true $= -0.1$, tau.true $= -0.5$, prob.cens $= 0\%$, $V \sim N(0,1)$, size $= 500$

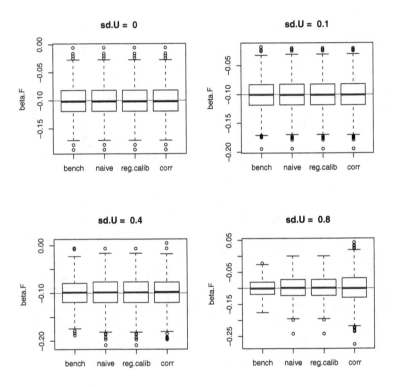

Figure C.29.: Boxplot for β_F with beta.V.true = 0.6, beta.F.true = -0.1, tau.true = -0.5, prob.cens = 0%, $V \sim N(0,1)$, size = 500

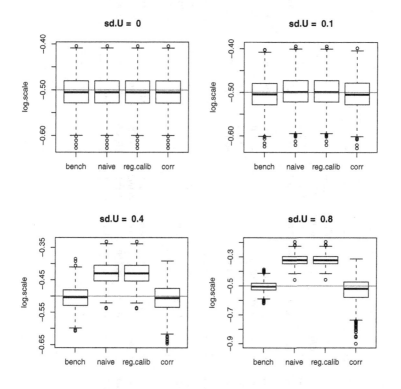

Figure C.30.: Boxplot for τ with beta.V.true $= 0.6$, beta.F.true $= -0.1$, tau.true $=$ -0.5, prob.cens $= 0\%$, $V \sim N(0,1)$, size $= 500$

	$\hat{\beta}_V$	$med(\hat{\beta}_V)$	$sd(\hat{\beta}_V)$	$sd(\hat{\beta}_V)$	$\% \in$ CI	$\widehat{MSE}$	$\hat{\beta}_F$	$med(\hat{\beta}_F)$	$sd(\hat{\beta}_F)$	$sd(\hat{\beta}_F)$	$\% \in$ CI	$\widehat{MSE}$	$\widehat{E(T)}$
sd.U = 0													
benchmark	0.599	0.600	0.026	0.027	95.200	0.001	-0.100	-0.101	0.027	0.027	94.900	0.001	0.894
naive	0.599	0.600	0.026	0.027	95.200	0.001	-0.100	-0.101	0.027	0.027	94.900	0.001	0.894
reg.calib	0.599	0.600	0.026	0.027	95.200	0.001	-0.100	-0.101	0.027	0.027	94.900	0.001	0.894
corr	0.599	0.600	0.026	0.027	95.300	0.001	-0.100	-0.101	0.027	0.027	94.300	0.001	0.894
sd.U = 0.1													
benchmark	0.600	0.599	0.027	0.027	95.100	0.001	-0.101	-0.101	0.028	0.027	93.600	0.001	0.896
naive	0.594	0.593	0.027	0.027	95.000	0.001	-0.101	-0.101	0.028	0.027	93.500	0.001	0.896
reg.calib	0.600	0.599	0.028	0.027	95.100	0.001	-0.101	-0.101	0.028	0.027	93.500	0.001	0.896
corr	0.600	0.600	0.028	0.027	94.800	0.001	-0.101	-0.101	0.028	0.027	93.700	0.001	0.896
sd.U = 0.4													
benchmark	0.601	0.602	0.027	0.027	95.100	0.001	-0.099	-0.099	0.028	0.027	94.800	0.001	0.895
naive	0.518	0.519	0.029	0.027	15.400	0.008	-0.099	-0.099	0.031	0.029	94.400	0.001	0.901
reg.calib	0.601	0.603	0.034	0.032	92.300	0.001	-0.099	-0.099	0.031	0.029	94.400	0.001	0.901
corr	0.603	0.604	0.036	0.034	93.000	0.001	-0.099	-0.098	0.032	0.031	94.400	0.001	0.894
sd.U = 0.8													
benchmark	0.600	0.600	0.028	0.027	95.200	0.001	-0.100	-0.101	0.028	0.027	94.500	0.001	0.893
naive	0.366	0.366	0.029	0.026	0.000	0.056	-0.099	-0.099	0.036	0.033	92.500	0.001	0.913
reg.calib	0.603	0.602	0.054	0.042	86.900	0.003	-0.099	-0.099	0.036	0.033	92.500	0.001	0.913
corr	0.616	0.610	0.070	0.067	96.509	0.005	-0.100	-0.100	0.046	0.042	92.505	0.002	0.892

Table C.15.: Results for β_V and β_F with beta.V.true = 0.6, beta.F.true = -0.1, tau.true = -0.5, prob.cens = 0%, $V \sim N(0,1)$ and size = 500

	$\bar{\hat{\tau}}$	$med(\hat{\tau})$	$sd(\hat{\tau})$	$\overline{sd(\hat{\tau})}$	$\% \in$ CI	$\widehat{MSE}$	#NA
sd.U $= 0$							
benchmark	-0.505	-0.505	0.035	0.035	95.300	0.001	0
naive	-0.505	-0.505	0.035	0.035	95.300	0.001	0
reg.calib	-0.505	-0.505	0.035	0.035	95.300	0.001	0
corr	-0.505	-0.505	0.035	0.035	95.000	0.001	0
sd.U $= 0.1$							
benchmark1	-0.504	-0.504	0.036	0.035	94.800	0.001	0
naive1	-0.498	-0.499	0.036	0.035	94.700	0.001	0
reg.calib1	-0.498	-0.499	0.036	0.035	94.700	0.001	0
corr1	-0.504	-0.505	0.036	0.035	94.600	0.001	0
sd.U $= 0.4$							
benchmark2	-0.504	-0.503	0.035	0.035	94.600	0.001	0
naive2	-0.430	-0.430	0.034	0.034	46.500	0.006	0
reg.calib2	-0.430	-0.430	0.034	0.034	46.500	0.006	0
corr2	-0.507	-0.506	0.042	0.042	94.700	0.002	0
sd.U $= 0.8$							
benchmark3	-0.505	-0.504	0.036	0.035	93.600	0.001	0
naive3	-0.321	-0.323	0.036	0.034	0.100	0.033	0
reg.calib3	-0.321	-0.323	0.036	0.034	0.100	0.033	0
corr3	-0.530	-0.519	0.089	0.083	97.125	0.009	26

Table C.16.: Results for τ with beta.V.true $= 0.6$, beta.F.true $= -0.1$, tau.true $=$ -0.5, prob.cens $= 0\%$, $V \sim N(0,1)$ and size $= 500$

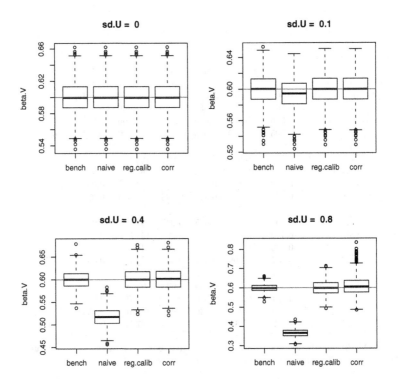

Figure C.31.: Boxplot for β_V with beta.V.true = 0.6, beta.F.true = -0.1, tau.true = -0.5, prob.cens = 0%, $V \sim N(0,1)$, size = 1000

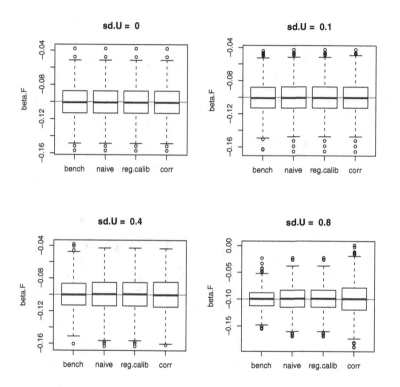

Figure C.32.: Boxplot for β_F with `beta.V.true` = 0.6, `beta.F.true` = -0.1, `tau.true` = -0.5, `prob.cens` = 0%, $V \sim N(0,1)$, `size` = 1000

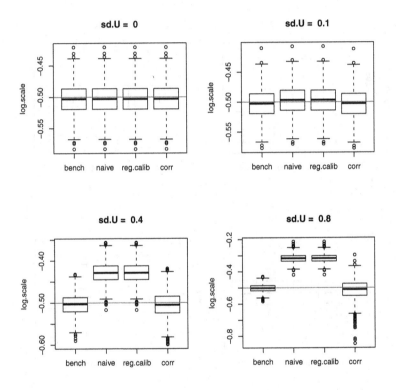

Figure C.33.: Boxplot for τ with beta.V.true $= 0.6$, beta.F.true $= -0.1$, tau.true $=$ -0.5, prob.cens $= 0\%$, $V \sim N(0,1)$, size $= 1000$

	$\hat{\beta}_V$	$med(\hat{\beta}_V)$	$sd(\hat{\beta}_V)$	$sd(\widehat{\hat{\beta}_V})$	$\% \in$ CI	$\widehat{MSE}$	$\hat{\beta}_F$	$med(\hat{\beta}_F)$	$sd(\hat{\beta}_F)$	$sd(\widehat{\hat{\beta}_F})$	$\% \in$ CI	$\widehat{MSE}$	$\widehat{\mathbb{E}(T)}$
sd.U = 0													
benchmark	0.600	0.600	0.020	0.019	94.900	0.000	-0.100	-0.101	0.019	0.019	95.900	0.000	0.894
naive	0.600	0.600	0.020	0.019	94.900	0.000	-0.100	-0.101	0.019	0.019	95.900	0.000	0.894
reg.calib	0.600	0.600	0.020	0.019	94.900	0.000	-0.100	-0.101	0.019	0.019	95.900	0.000	0.894
corr	0.600	0.600	0.020	0.019	94.900	0.000	-0.100	-0.101	0.019	0.019	96.100	0.000	0.894
sd.U = 0.1													
benchmark	0.600	0.600	0.019	0.019	95.900	0.000	-0.101	-0.101	0.019	0.019	94.800	0.000	0.895
naive	0.594	0.594	0.019	0.019	94.600	0.000	-0.100	-0.101	0.019	0.019	95.000	0.000	0.895
reg.calib	0.600	0.600	0.019	0.019	95.800	0.000	-0.100	-0.101	0.019	0.019	95.000	0.000	0.895
corr	0.600	0.600	0.019	0.019	95.600	0.000	-0.100	-0.100	0.019	0.019	94.200	0.000	0.895
sd.U = 0.4													
benchmark	0.600	0.600	0.019	0.019	94.000	0.000	-0.100	-0.100	0.019	0.019	95.100	0.000	0.895
naive	0.517	0.517	0.021	0.019	1.100	0.007	-0.100	-0.100	0.021	0.021	94.500	0.000	0.901
reg.calib	0.600	0.600	0.024	0.022	93.100	0.001	-0.100	-0.100	0.021	0.021	94.500	0.000	0.902
corr	0.601	0.601	0.025	0.024	93.900	0.001	-0.099	-0.100	0.022	0.022	95.200	0.000	0.895
sd.U = 0.8													
benchmark	0.599	0.599	0.020	0.019	94.500	0.000	-0.099	-0.099	0.019	0.019	95.400	0.000	0.894
naive	0.365	0.365	0.020	0.018	0.000	0.056	-0.099	-0.099	0.024	0.023	94.100	0.001	0.914
reg.calib	0.600	0.599	0.038	0.030	88.500	0.001	-0.099	-0.099	0.024	0.023	94.100	0.001	0.914
corr	0.609	0.606	0.050	0.046	95.000	0.003	-0.099	-0.100	0.031	0.030	93.800	0.001	0.894

Table C.17.: Results for β_V and β_F with beta.V.true = 0.6, beta.F.true = -0.1, tau.true = -0.5, prob.cens = 0%, $V \sim N(0,1)$ and size = 1000

	$\bar{\hat{\tau}}$	$med(\hat{\tau})$	$sd(\hat{\tau})$	$\overline{sd(\hat{\tau})}$	$\% \in$ CI	$\widehat{MSE}$	#NA
sd.U $= 0$							
benchmark	-0.503	-0.503	0.024	0.025	95.600	0.001	0
naive	-0.503	-0.503	0.024	0.025	95.600	0.001	0
reg.calib	-0.503	-0.503	0.024	0.025	95.600	0.001	0
corr	-0.503	-0.503	0.024	0.025	95.600	0.001	0
sd.U $= 0.1$							
benchmark	-0.503	-0.502	0.024	0.025	96.300	0.001	0
naive	-0.497	-0.497	0.024	0.025	96.000	0.001	0
reg.calib	-0.497	-0.497	0.024	0.025	96.000	0.001	0
corr	-0.503	-0.502	0.024	0.025	96.300	0.001	0
sd.U $= 0.4$							
benchmark	-0.503	-0.503	0.025	0.025	95.000	0.001	0
naive	-0.428	-0.429	0.025	0.024	15.800	0.006	0
reg.calib	-0.428	-0.429	0.025	0.024	15.800	0.006	0
corr	-0.505	-0.505	0.030	0.030	94.500	0.001	0
sd.U $= 0.8$							
benchmark	-0.501	-0.501	0.024	0.025	94.000	0.001	0
naive	-0.318	-0.317	0.027	0.024	0.000	0.034	0
reg.calib	-0.318	-0.317	0.027	0.024	0.000	0.034	0
corr	-0.516	-0.510	0.063	0.055	93.800	0.004	0

Table C.18.: Results for τ with beta.V.true $= 0.6$, beta.F.true $= -0.1$, tau.true $=$ -0.5, prob.cens $= 0\%$, $V \sim N(0,1)$ and size $= 1000$

C.2.2. beta.V.true = 0.6, beta.F.true = -0.1 , tau.true = -0.5, prob.cens = 0% and $V \sim Unif(0, \sqrt{12})$

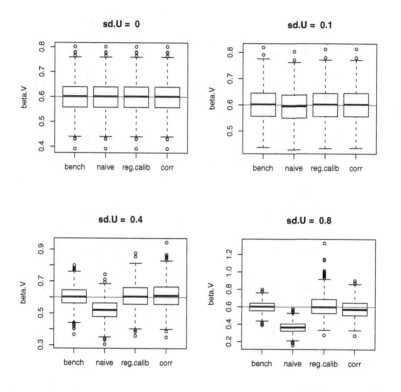

Figure C.34.: Boxplot for β_V with beta.V.true = 0.6, beta.F.true = -0.1, tau.true = -0.5, prob.cens = 0%, $V \sim Unif(0, \sqrt{12})$, size = 100

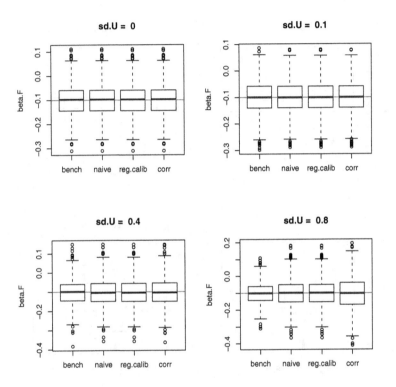

Figure C.35.: Boxplot for β_F with beta.V.true = 0.6, beta.F.true = -0.1, tau.true = -0.5, prob.cens = 0%, $V \sim Unif(0, \sqrt{12})$, size = 100

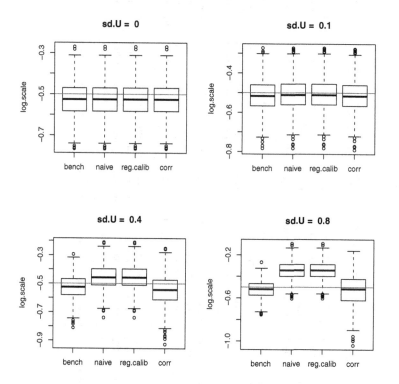

Figure C.36.: Boxplot for τ with beta.V.true $= 0.6$, beta.F.true $= -0.1$, tau.true $=$ -0.5, prob.cens $= 0\%$, $V \sim Unif(0, \sqrt{12})$, size $= 100$

	$\hat{\beta}_V$	$med(\hat{\beta}_V)$	$sd(\hat{\beta}_V)$	$sd(\hat{\beta}_V)$	$\% \in CI$	$\widehat{MSE}$	$\hat{\beta}_F$	$med(\hat{\beta}_F)$	$sd(\hat{\beta}_F)$	$sd(\hat{\beta}_F)$	$\% \in CI$	$\widehat{MSE}$	$\mathbb{E}(T)$
sd.U = 0													
benchmark	0.600	0.601	0.062	0.061	94.000	0.004	-0.101	-0.098	0.064	0.062	93.800	0.004	2.552
naive	0.600	0.601	0.062	0.061	94.000	0.004	-0.101	-0.098	0.064	0.062	93.800	0.004	2.552
reg.calib	0.600	0.601	0.062	0.061	94.000	0.004	-0.101	-0.098	0.064	0.062	93.800	0.004	2.552
corr	0.600	0.601	0.062	0.059	92.700	0.004	-0.101	-0.098	0.064	0.058	91.900	0.004	2.552
sd.U = 0.1													
benchmark	0.602	0.602	0.061	0.061	95.900	0.004	-0.100	-0.100	0.061	0.062	95.000	0.004	2.561
naive	0.596	0.596	0.060	0.062	95.700	0.004	-0.100	-0.100	0.062	0.062	95.000	0.004	2.535
reg.calib	0.602	0.602	0.061	0.062	95.700	0.004	-0.100	-0.100	0.062	0.062	95.000	0.004	2.562
corr	0.603	0.602	0.061	0.060	94.900	0.004	-0.099	-0.100	0.062	0.059	93.800	0.004	2.562
sd.U = 0.4													
benchmark	0.602	0.603	0.061	0.061	95.100	0.004	-0.100	-0.099	0.065	0.061	93.500	0.004	2.552
naive	0.521	0.521	0.063	0.061	73.000	0.010	-0.101	-0.103	0.070	0.066	93.800	0.005	2.236
reg.calib	0.606	0.604	0.077	0.071	92.900	0.006	-0.101	-0.103	0.070	0.066	93.800	0.005	2.599
corr	0.613	0.610	0.081	0.072	91.400	0.007	-0.102	-0.104	0.072	0.065	91.300	0.005	2.616
sd.U = 0.8													
benchmark	0.600	0.603	0.064	0.061	93.500	0.004	-0.101	-0.101	0.063	0.062	94.400	0.004	2.553
naive	0.365	0.364	0.061	0.058	2.900	0.059	-0.100	-0.099	0.081	0.074	91.800	0.007	1.728
reg.calib	0.609	0.599	0.122	0.097	88.700	0.015	-0.100	-0.099	0.081	0.074	91.800	0.007	2.690
corr	0.576	0.570	0.104	0.224	93.617	0.011	-0.104	-0.102	0.100	0.104	91.337	0.010	2.482

Table C.19.: Results for β_V and β_F with beta.V.true = 0.6, beta.F.true = -0.1, tau.true = -0.5, prob.cens = 0%, $V \sim Unif(0, \sqrt{12})$ and size = 100

	$\bar{\hat{\tau}}$	$med(\hat{\tau})$	$sd(\hat{\tau})$	$\overline{sd(\hat{\tau})}$	$\% \in$ CI	$\widehat{MSE}$	#NA
sd.U $= 0$							
benchmark	-0.526	-0.525	0.081	0.078	93.300	0.007	0
naive	-0.526	-0.525	0.081	0.078	93.300	0.007	0
reg.calib	-0.526	-0.525	0.081	0.078	93.300	0.007	0
corr	-0.526	-0.525	0.081	0.076	91.900	0.007	0
sd.U $= 0.1$							
benchmark	-0.516	-0.516	0.078	0.078	95.100	0.006	0
naive	-0.510	-0.511	0.078	0.078	95.000	0.006	0
reg.calib	-0.510	-0.511	0.078	0.078	95.000	0.006	0
corr	-0.517	-0.517	0.079	0.077	94.000	0.007	0
sd.U $= 0.4$							
benchmark	-0.528	-0.525	0.082	0.078	92.600	0.007	0
naive	-0.456	-0.458	0.083	0.078	88.800	0.009	0
reg.calib	-0.456	-0.458	0.083	0.078	88.800	0.009	0
corr	-0.546	-0.544	0.105	0.094	90.300	0.013	0
sd.U $= 0.8$							
benchmark	-0.521	-0.518	0.078	0.078	94.400	0.007	0
naive	-0.346	-0.343	0.081	0.076	46.500	0.030	0
reg.calib	-0.346	-0.343	0.081	0.076	46.500	0.030	0
corr	-0.529	-0.516	0.141	0.212	96.809	0.021	342

Table C.20.: Results for τ with beta.V.true $= 0.6$, beta.F.true $= -0.1$, tau.true $= -0.5$, prob.cens $= 0\%$, $V \sim Unif(0, \sqrt{12})$ and size $= 100$

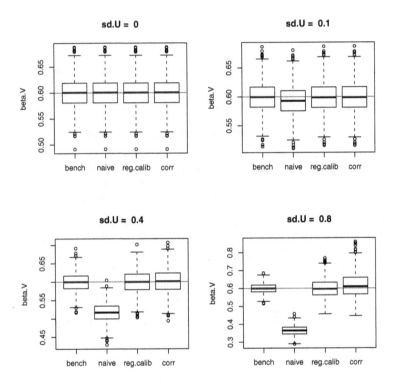

Figure C.37.: Boxplot for β_V with beta.V.true = 0.6, beta.F.true = -0.1, tau.true
= -0.5, prob.cens = 0%, $V \sim Unif(0, \sqrt{12})$, size = 500

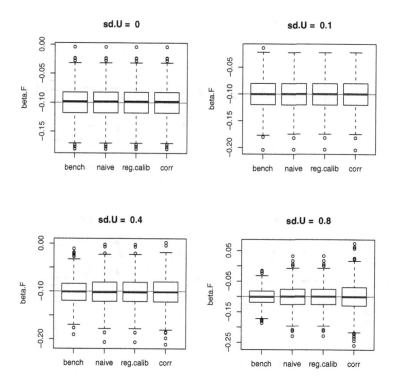

Figure C.38.: Boxplot for β_F with `beta.V.true` = 0.6, `beta.F.true` = -0.1, `tau.true` = -0.5, `prob.cens` = 0%, $V \sim Unif(0, \sqrt{12})$, `size` = 500

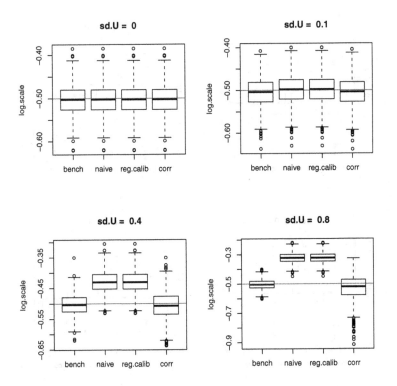

Figure C.39.: Boxplot for τ with beta.V.true = 0.6, beta.F.true = -0.1, tau.true = -0.5, prob.cens = 0%, $V \sim Unif(0, \sqrt{12})$, size = 500

	$\hat{\beta}_V$	$med(\hat{\beta}_V)$	$sd(\hat{\beta}_V)$	$\widetilde{sd}(\hat{\beta}_V)$	$\% \in CI$	$\widehat{MSE}$	$\hat{\beta}_F$	$med(\hat{\beta}_F)$	$sd(\hat{\beta}_F)$	$\widetilde{sd}(\hat{\beta}_F)$	$\% \in CI$	$\widehat{MSE}$	$\widehat{\mathbb{E}(T)}$
sd.U = 0													
benchmark	0.600	0.600	0.028	0.027	94.700	0.001	-0.100	-0.098	0.027	0.027	94.500	0.001	2.531
naive	0.600	0.600	0.028	0.027	94.700	0.001	-0.100	-0.098	0.027	0.027	94.500	0.001	2.531
reg.calib	0.600	0.600	0.028	0.027	94.700	0.001	-0.100	-0.098	0.027	0.027	94.500	0.001	2.531
corr	0.600	0.600	0.028	0.027	94.200	0.001	-0.100	-0.098	0.027	0.027	94.100	0.001	2.531
sd.U = 0.1													
benchmark	0.599	0.600	0.027	0.027	95.700	0.001	-0.100	-0.100	0.028	0.027	94.800	0.001	2.527
naive	0.593	0.593	0.027	0.027	94.400	0.001	-0.100	-0.100	0.028	0.027	94.900	0.001	2.501
reg.calib	0.599	0.599	0.027	0.027	95.200	0.001	-0.100	-0.100	0.028	0.027	94.900	0.001	2.527
corr	0.599	0.599	0.027	0.027	94.800	0.001	-0.100	-0.100	0.028	0.027	94.400	0.001	2.526
sd.U = 0.4													
benchmark	0.600	0.600	0.026	0.027	95.900	0.001	-0.101	-0.101	0.027	0.027	96.100	0.001	2.529
naive	0.517	0.517	0.027	0.027	13.000	0.008	-0.100	-0.102	0.030	0.029	94.400	0.001	2.206
reg.calib	0.600	0.600	0.032	0.032	94.900	0.001	-0.100	-0.102	0.030	0.029	94.400	0.001	2.549
corr	0.601	0.601	0.033	0.034	94.700	0.001	-0.101	-0.101	0.031	0.030	94.400	0.001	2.538
sd.U = 0.8													
benchmark	0.599	0.599	0.028	0.027	94.400	0.001	-0.100	-0.101	0.027	0.027	95.200	0.001	2.529
naive	0.363	0.363	0.027	0.026	0.000	0.057	-0.100	-0.099	0.036	0.033	93.300	0.001	1.715
reg.calib	0.599	0.597	0.053	0.043	88.600	0.003	-0.100	-0.099	0.036	0.033	93.300	0.001	2.588
corr	0.615	0.609	0.068	0.067	96.917	0.005	-0.101	-0.101	0.045	0.042	92.806	0.002	2.611

Table C.21.: Results for β_V and β_F with beta.V.true = 0.6, beta.F.true = -0.1, tau.true = -0.5, prob.cens = 0%, $V \sim Unif(0, \sqrt{12})$ and size = 500

	$\bar{\hat{\tau}}$	$med(\hat{\tau})$	$sd(\hat{\tau})$	$\overline{sd(\hat{\tau})}$	$\% \in$ CI	$\widehat{MSE}$	#NA
sd.U $= 0$							
benchmark	-0.503	-0.503	0.034	0.035	95.400	0.001	0
naive	-0.503	-0.503	0.034	0.035	95.400	0.001	0
reg.calib	-0.503	-0.503	0.034	0.035	95.400	0.001	0
corr	-0.503	-0.503	0.034	0.035	95.300	0.001	0
sd.U $= 0.1$							
benchmark1	-0.504	-0.504	0.035	0.035	95.200	0.001	0
naive1	-0.498	-0.498	0.035	0.035	95.100	0.001	0
reg.calib1	-0.498	-0.498	0.035	0.035	95.100	0.001	0
corr1	-0.504	-0.504	0.035	0.035	95.000	0.001	0
sd.U $= 0.4$							
benchmark2	-0.502	-0.504	0.034	0.035	95.200	0.001	0
naive2	-0.429	-0.430	0.035	0.034	47.500	0.006	0
reg.calib2	-0.429	-0.430	0.035	0.034	47.500	0.006	0
corr2	-0.506	-0.508	0.042	0.042	94.300	0.002	0
sd.U $= 0.8$							
benchmark3	-0.505	-0.504	0.034	0.035	95.200	0.001	0
naive3	-0.323	-0.323	0.036	0.034	0.100	0.033	0
reg.calib3	-0.323	-0.323	0.036	0.034	0.100	0.033	0
corr3	-0.531	-0.521	0.085	0.083	96.814	0.008	27

Table C.22.: Results for τ with beta.V.true $= 0.6$, beta.F.true $= -0.1$, tau.true $= -0.5$, prob.cens $= 0\%$, $V \sim Unif(0, \sqrt{12})$ and size $= 500$

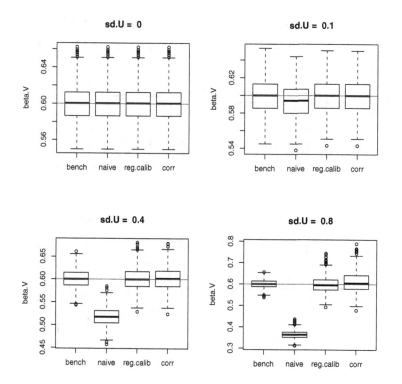

Figure C.40.: Boxplot for β_V with beta.V.true $= 0.6$, beta.F.true $= -0.1$, tau.true $= -0.5$, prob.cens $= 0\%$, $V \sim Unif(0, \sqrt{12})$, size $= 1000$

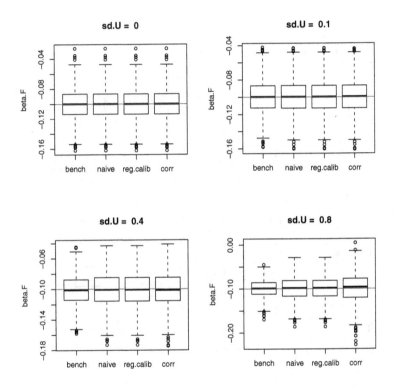

Figure C.41.: Boxplot for β_F with beta.V.true = 0.6, beta.F.true = -0.1, tau.true = -0.5, prob.cens = 0%, $V \sim Unif(0, \sqrt{12})$, size = 1000

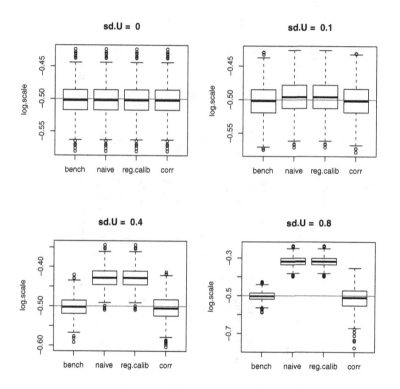

Figure C.42.: Boxplot for τ with beta.V.true $= 0.6$, beta.F.true $= -0.1$, tau.true $=$ -0.5, prob.cens $= 0\%$, $V \sim Unif(0, \sqrt{12})$, size $= 1000$

	$\hat{\beta}_V$	$med(\hat{\beta}_V)$	$sd(\hat{\beta}_V)$	$sd(\hat{\beta}_V)$	$\% \in CI$	$\widehat{MSE}$	$\hat{\beta}_F$	$med(\hat{\beta}_F)$	$sd(\hat{\beta}_F)$	$sd(\hat{\beta}_F)$	$\% \in CI$	$\widehat{MSE}$	$\widehat{\mathbb{E}(T)}$
sd.U = 0													
benchmark	0.600	0.600	0.019	0.019	95.100	0.000	-0.100	-0.100	0.020	0.019	94.600	0.000	2.535
naive	0.600	0.600	0.019	0.019	95.100	0.000	-0.100	-0.100	0.020	0.019	94.600	0.000	2.535
reg.calib	0.600	0.600	0.019	0.019	95.100	0.000	-0.100	-0.100	0.020	0.019	94.600	0.000	2.535
corr	0.600	0.600	0.019	0.019	94.900	0.000	-0.100	-0.100	0.020	0.019	93.700	0.000	2.535
sd.U = 0.1													
benchmark	0.600	0.600	0.019	0.019	95.700	0.000	-0.100	-0.100	0.020	0.019	93.300	0.000	2.527
naive	0.593	0.594	0.019	0.019	94.300	0.000	-0.100	-0.100	0.020	0.019	92.600	0.000	2.501
reg.calib	0.599	0.600	0.019	0.019	96.000	0.000	-0.100	-0.100	0.020	0.019	92.600	0.000	2.527
corr	0.599	0.600	0.019	0.019	96.000	0.000	-0.100	-0.100	0.020	0.019	92.200	0.000	2.526
sd.U = 0.4													
benchmark	0.601	0.600	0.019	0.019	94.700	0.000	-0.101	-0.101	0.020	0.019	93.500	0.000	2.536
naive	0.518	0.518	0.020	0.019	1.300	0.007	-0.101	-0.101	0.022	0.021	93.000	0.001	2.213
reg.calib	0.601	0.600	0.023	0.022	95.300	0.001	-0.101	-0.101	0.022	0.021	93.000	0.001	2.556
corr	0.602	0.602	0.024	0.024	95.200	0.001	-0.101	-0.101	0.023	0.022	93.700	0.001	2.542
sd.U = 0.8													
benchmark	0.601	0.600	0.019	0.019	94.400	0.000	-0.099	-0.099	0.019	0.019	94.800	0.000	2.532
naive	0.364	0.364	0.019	0.018	0.000	0.056	-0.099	-0.098	0.025	0.023	93.300	0.001	1.717
reg.calib	0.598	0.596	0.036	0.030	89.900	0.001	-0.099	-0.098	0.025	0.023	93.300	0.001	2.578
corr	0.610	0.605	0.047	0.046	96.181	0.002	-0.098	-0.097	0.033	0.030	92.764	0.001	2.579

Table C.23.: Results for β_V and β_F with beta.V.true = 0.6, beta.F.true = -0.1, tau.true = -0.5, prob.cens = 0%, $V \sim Unif(0, \sqrt{12})$ and size = 1000

	$\bar{\hat{\tau}}$	$med(\hat{\tau})$	$sd(\hat{\tau})$	$\overline{sd(\hat{\tau})}$	$\% \in$ CI	$\widehat{MSE}$	#NA
sd.U $= 0$							
benchmark	-0.502	-0.502	0.024	0.025	95.600	0.001	0
naive	-0.502	-0.502	0.024	0.025	95.600	0.001	0
reg.calib	-0.502	-0.502	0.024	0.025	95.600	0.001	0
corr	-0.502	-0.502	0.024	0.025	95.500	0.001	0
sd.U $= 0.1$							
benchmark	-0.502	-0.502	0.026	0.025	93.300	0.001	0
naive	-0.496	-0.496	0.025	0.025	93.300	0.001	0
reg.calib	-0.496	-0.496	0.025	0.025	93.300	0.001	0
corr	-0.502	-0.502	0.026	0.025	94.000	0.001	0
sd.U $= 0.4$							
benchmark	-0.502	-0.502	0.025	0.025	94.900	0.001	0
naive	-0.427	-0.428	0.025	0.024	16.100	0.006	0
reg.calib	-0.427	-0.428	0.025	0.024	16.100	0.006	0
corr	-0.504	-0.505	0.031	0.030	94.200	0.001	0
sd.U $= 0.8$							
benchmark	-0.502	-0.502	0.025	0.025	93.600	0.001	0
naive	-0.319	-0.319	0.026	0.024	0.000	0.034	0
reg.calib	-0.319	-0.319	0.026	0.024	0.000	0.034	0
corr	-0.515	-0.510	0.060	0.055	95.477	0.004	5

Table C.24.: Results for τ with beta.V.true $= 0.6$, beta.F.true $= -0.1$, tau.true $=$ -0.5, prob.cens $= 0\%$, $V \sim Unif(0, \sqrt{12})$ and size $= 1000$

C.3. Structural Changes - single

C.3.1. beta.1.true = 0.6, beta.2.true = -0.2 , tau.1.true = 0.5, tau.2.true = -0.4, prob.cens = 35% and $V \sim N(0, 1)$

	%#mob	#mob	not #mob	#NA
sd.U = 0				
benchmark	92.0	460	40	0
naive	92.0	460	40	0
reg.calib	92.0	460	40	0
corr	92.0	460	40	0
sd.U = 0.1				
benchmark	91.2	456	44	0
naive	90.6	453	47	0
reg.calib	90.6	453	47	0
corr	90.4	452	48	0
sd.U = 0.4				
benchmark	91.8	459	41	0
naive	91.4	457	43	0
reg.calib	91.4	457	43	0
corr	91.2	456	44	0
sd.U = 0.8				
benchmark	92.8	464	36	0
naive	88.2	441	59	0
reg.calib	88.2	441	59	0
corr	70.2	351	149	82

Table C.25.: Detection of the true structural change with beta.1.true = 0.6, beta.2.true = -0.2 , tau.1.true = 0.5, tau.2.true = -0.4, prob.cens = 35%, $V \sim N(0, 1)$ and size = 100

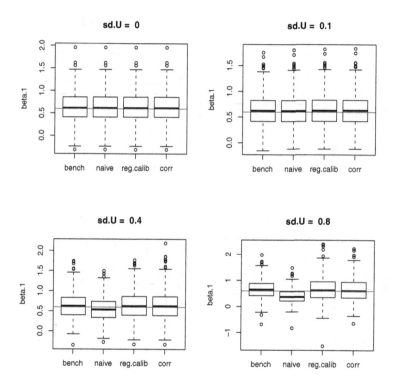

Figure C.43.: Boxplot for β_1 with beta.1.true $= 0.6$, beta.2.true $= -0.2$, tau.1.true $= 0.5$, tau.2.true $= -0.4$, prob.cens $= 35\%$, $V \sim N(0,1)$, size $= 100$

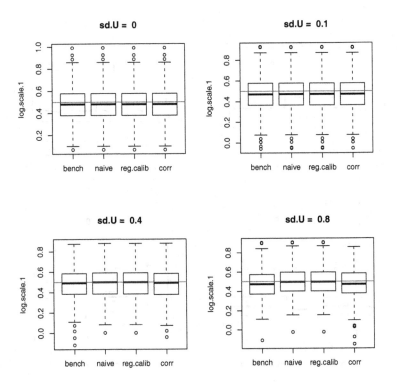

Figure C.44.: Boxplot for τ_1 with beta.1.true = 0.6, beta.2.true = -0.2 , tau.1.true
= 0.5, tau.2.true = -0.4, prob.cens = 35%, $V \sim N(0,1)$, size = 100

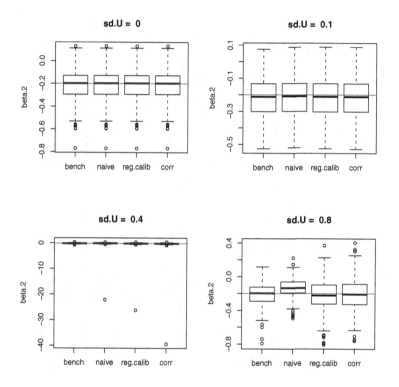

Figure C.45.: Boxplot for β_2 with beta.1.true $= 0.6$, beta.2.true $= -0.2$, tau.1.true $= 0.5$, tau.2.true $= -0.4$, prob.cens $= 35\%$, $V \sim N(0,1)$, size $= 100$

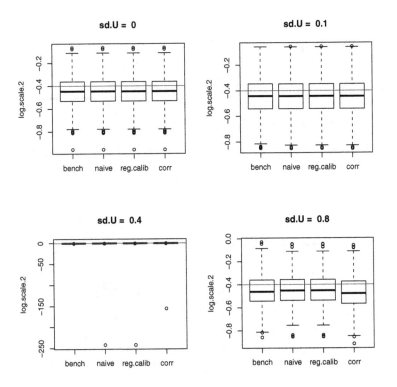

Figure C.46.: Boxplot for τ_2 with `beta.1.true` = 0.6, `beta.2.true` = -0.2, `tau.1.true` = 0.5, `tau.2.true` = -0.4, `prob.cens` = 35%, $V \sim N(0,1)$, `size` = 100

	$\hat{\bar{\beta}}_1$	$med(\hat{\beta}_1)$	$sd(\hat{\beta}_1)$	$\overline{sd(\hat{\beta}_1)}$	$\% \in CI$	$\widehat{MSE}$	$\widehat{\mathbb{E}(T)}$	$\hat{\bar{\tau}}_1$	$med(\hat{\tau}_1)$	$sd(\hat{\tau}_1)$	$\overline{sd(\hat{\tau}_1)}$	$\% \in CI$	$\widehat{MSE}$
sd.U = 0													
benchmark	0.626	0.613	0.324	0.319	95.217	0.106	1.521	0.480	0.480	0.146	0.152	95.652	0.022
naive	0.626	0.613	0.324	0.319	95.217	0.106	1.521	0.480	0.480	0.146	0.152	95.652	0.022
reg.calib	0.626	0.613	0.324	0.319	95.217	0.106	1.521	0.480	0.480	0.146	0.152	95.652	0.022
corr	0.626	0.613	0.324	0.313	95.000	0.106	1.521	0.480	0.480	0.146	0.148	94.130	0.022
sd.U = 0.1													
benchmark	0.636	0.627	0.308	0.314	95.175	0.096	1.514	0.472	0.471	0.162	0.151	93.202	0.027
naive	0.630	0.624	0.307	0.313	94.923	0.095	1.515	0.473	0.472	0.162	0.151	93.598	0.027
reg.calib	0.637	0.628	0.310	0.316	95.143	0.097	1.515	0.473	0.472	0.162	0.151	93.598	0.027
corr	0.638	0.632	0.312	0.310	93.142	0.098	1.514	0.473	0.472	0.162	0.147	92.699	0.027
sd.U = 0.4													
benchmark	0.632	0.626	0.317	0.315	96.950	0.101	1.518	0.482	0.491	0.151	0.151	95.425	0.023
naive	0.550	0.537	0.306	0.295	93.654	0.096	1.531	0.489	0.498	0.149	0.152	95.842	0.022
reg.calib	0.641	0.625	0.359	0.344	96.061	0.130	1.531	0.489	0.498	0.149	0.152	95.842	0.022
corr	0.654	0.626	0.382	0.349	94.518	0.148	1.513	0.478	0.491	0.153	0.149	93.202	0.024
sd.U = 0.8													
benchmark	0.658	0.647	0.348	0.321	95.043	0.124	1.507	0.475	0.473	0.145	0.152	96.336	0.022
naive	0.397	0.376	0.273	0.253	85.261	0.116	1.552	0.496	0.497	0.146	0.152	96.372	0.021
reg.calib	0.665	0.631	0.466	0.429	94.558	0.221	1.553	0.496	0.497	0.146	0.152	96.372	0.021
corr	0.660	0.607	0.465	0.633	97.436	0.219	1.512	0.471	0.472	0.157	0.172	94.872	0.025

Table C.26.: Results for node 2 with beta.1.true $= 0.6$, beta.2.true $= -0.2$, tau.1.true $= 0.5$, tau.2.true $= -0.4$, prob.cens $= 35\%$, $V \sim N(0,1)$ and size $= 100$

	$\hat{\bar{\beta}}_2$	$med(\hat{\beta}_2)$	$sd(\hat{\beta}_2)$	$\widehat{sd}(\hat{\beta}_2)$	$\% \in CI$	$\widehat{MSE}$	$\widehat{E}(T)$	$\hat{\bar{\tau}}_2$	$med(\hat{\tau}_2)$	$sd(\hat{\tau}_2)$	$\widehat{sd}(\hat{\tau}_2)$	$\% \in CI$	$\widehat{MSE}$
sd.U = 0													
benchmark	-0.209	-0.199	0.127	0.121	93.478	0.016	0.903	-0.448	-0.446	0.132	0.137	94.348	0.020
naive	-0.209	-0.199	0.127	0.121	93.478	0.016	0.903	-0.448	-0.446	0.132	0.137	94.348	0.020
reg.calib	-0.209	-0.199	0.127	0.121	93.478	0.016	0.903	-0.448	-0.446	0.132	0.137	94.348	0.020
corr	-0.209	-0.199	0.127	0.116	90.870	0.016	0.903	-0.448	-0.446	0.132	0.135	93.913	0.020
sd.U = 0.1													
benchmark	-0.216	-0.211	0.121	0.121	94.518	0.015	0.903	-0.446	-0.441	0.142	0.137	92.982	0.022
naive	-0.214	-0.208	0.120	0.120	94.260	0.015	0.903	-0.447	-0.442	0.141	0.137	93.157	0.022
reg.calib	-0.216	-0.210	0.121	0.121	94.260	0.015	0.903	-0.447	-0.442	0.141	0.137	93.157	0.022
corr	-0.217	-0.211	0.121	0.118	94.027	0.015	0.903	-0.448	-0.444	0.141	0.133	92.699	0.022
sd.U = 0.4													
benchmark	-0.201	-0.197	0.124	0.122	94.336	0.015	0.905	-0.445	-0.445	0.146	0.137	93.028	0.023
naive	-0.220	-0.166	1.034	0.113	93.654	1.068	0.906	-0.971	-0.443	11.324	0.137	92.998	128.276
reg.calib	-0.257	-0.196	1.225	0.132	94.748	1.501	0.906	-0.971	-0.443	11.324	0.137	92.998	128.276
corr	-0.292	-0.196	1.843	>8m	93.421	3.399	0.906	-0.793	-0.451	7.285	0.142	89.693	53.109
sd.U = 0.8													
benchmark	-0.206	-0.197	0.130	0.120	93.319	0.017	0.904	-0.452	-0.461	0.142	0.137	92.888	0.023
naive	-0.129	-0.133	0.104	0.094	81.859	0.016	0.904	-0.442	-0.451	0.141	0.137	94.331	0.022
reg.calib	-0.217	-0.221	0.178	0.159	92.744	0.032	0.904	-0.442	-0.451	0.141	0.137	94.331	0.022
corr	-0.209	-0.207	0.187	0.186	94.872	0.035	0.902	-0.472	-0.478	0.149	0.155	94.872	0.027

Table C.27.: Results for node 3 with beta.1.true = 0.6, beta.2.true = -0.2, tau.1.true = 0.5, tau.2.true = -0.4, prob.cens = 35%, $V \sim N(0,1)$ and size = 100

	%#mob	#mob	not #mob	#NA
sd.U = 0				
benchmark	100	500	0	0
naive	100	500	0	0
reg.calib	100	500	0	0
corr	100	500	0	0
sd.U = 0.1				
benchmark	100	500	0	0
naive	100	500	0	0
reg.calib	100	500	0	0
corr	100	500	0	0
sd.U = 0.4				
benchmark	100	500	0	0
naive	100	500	0	0
reg.calib	100	500	0	0
corr	100	500	0	0
sd.U = 0.8				
benchmark	100	500	0	0
naive	100	500	0	0
reg.calib	100	500	0	0
corr	100	500	0	0

Table C.28.: Detection of the true structural change with `beta.1.true` = 0.6, `beta.2.true` = -0.2 , `tau.1.true` = 0.5, `tau.2.true` = -0.4, `prob.cens` = 35%, $V \sim N(0,1)$ and `size` = 500

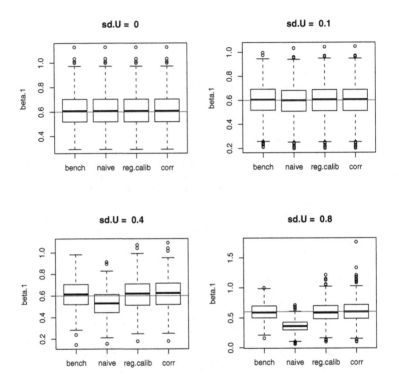

Figure C.47.: Boxplot for β_1 with beta.1.true $= 0.6$, beta.2.true $= -0.2$, tau.1.true $= 0.5$, tau.2.true $= -0.4$, prob.cens $= 35\%$, $V \sim N(0,1)$, size $= 500$

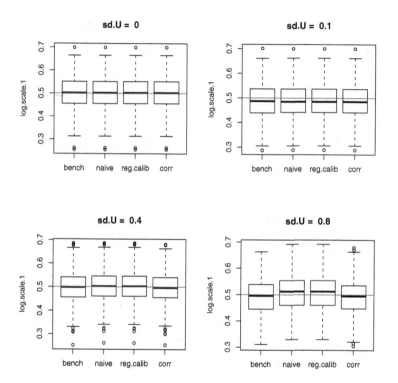

Figure C.48.: Boxplot for τ_1 with beta.1.true $= 0.6$, beta.2.true $= -0.2$, tau.1.true $= 0.5$, tau.2.true $= -0.4$, prob.cens $= 35\%$, $V \sim N(0,1)$, size $= 500$

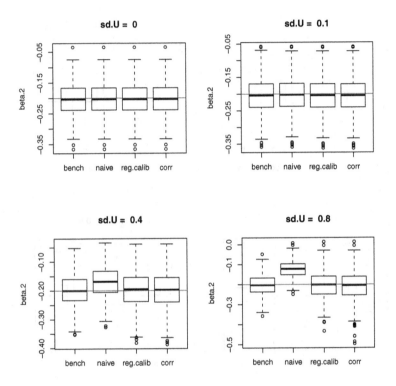

Figure C.49.: Boxplot for β_2 with beta.1.true = 0.6, beta.2.true = -0.2 , tau.1.true
= 0.5, tau.2.true = -0.4, prob.cens = 35%, $V \sim N(0, 1)$, size = 500

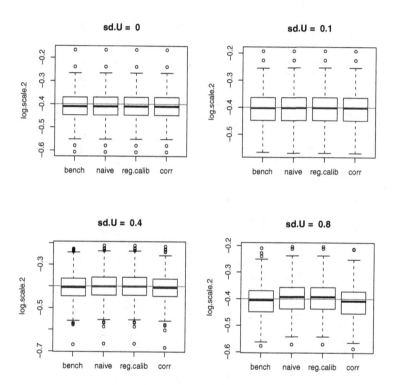

Figure C.50.: Boxplot for τ_2 with beta.1.true $= 0.6$, beta.2.true $= -0.2$, tau.1.true $= 0.5$, tau.2.true $= -0.4$, prob.cens $= 35\%$, $V \sim N(0,1)$, size $= 500$

	$\hat{\bar{\beta}}_1$	$med(\hat{\beta}_1)$	$sd(\hat{\beta}_1)$	$\overline{sd(\hat{\beta}_1)}$	$\% \in CI$	$\widehat{MSE}$	$\widehat{\mathbb{E}}(T)$	$\hat{\bar{\tau}}_1$	$med(\hat{\tau}_1)$	$sd(\hat{\tau}_1)$	$\overline{sd(\hat{\tau}_1)}$	$\% \in CI$	$\widehat{MSE}$
sd.U = 0													
benchmark	0.613	0.608	0.139	0.138	96.200	0.019	1.504	0.501	0.501	0.071	0.067	93.000	0.005
naive	0.613	0.608	0.139	0.138	96.200	0.019	1.504	0.501	0.501	0.071	0.067	93.000	0.005
reg.calib	0.613	0.608	0.139	0.138	96.200	0.019	1.504	0.501	0.501	0.071	0.067	93.000	0.005
corr	0.613	0.608	0.139	0.137	95.400	0.019	1.504	0.501	0.501	0.071	0.067	91.600	0.005
sd.U = 0.1													
benchmark	0.603	0.605	0.139	0.136	93.400	0.019	1.479	0.489	0.487	0.071	0.067	92.400	0.005
naive	0.597	0.600	0.139	0.136	93.400	0.019	1.480	0.490	0.486	0.071	0.067	92.400	0.005
reg.calib	0.603	0.606	0.140	0.137	93.400	0.020	1.480	0.490	0.486	0.071	0.067	92.400	0.005
corr	0.603	0.607	0.140	0.136	93.200	0.020	1.480	0.489	0.485	0.071	0.067	92.600	0.005
sd.U = 0.4													
benchmark	0.608	0.613	0.134	0.137	97.000	0.018	1.491	0.497	0.499	0.065	0.067	95.200	0.004
naive	0.527	0.529	0.122	0.128	89.200	0.020	1.501	0.502	0.503	0.065	0.067	95.400	0.004
reg.calib	0.612	0.619	0.142	0.148	96.800	0.020	1.501	0.502	0.503	0.065	0.067	95.400	0.004
corr	0.616	0.624	0.144	0.151	96.600	0.021	1.490	0.496	0.497	0.066	0.068	94.600	0.004
sd.U = 0.8													
benchmark	0.599	0.589	0.146	0.137	93.400	0.021	1.483	0.492	0.496	0.067	0.067	94.600	0.004
naive	0.359	0.356	0.107	0.106	36.200	0.069	1.511	0.507	0.512	0.066	0.067	95.200	0.004
reg.calib	0.591	0.584	0.177	0.175	94.200	0.031	1.511	0.507	0.512	0.066	0.067	95.200	0.004
corr	0.609	0.600	0.199	0.192	96.000	0.039	1.479	0.490	0.495	0.068	0.069	94.600	0.005

Table C.29.: Results for node 2 with beta.1.true = 0.6, beta.2.true = -0.2, tau.1.true = 0.5, tau.2.true = -0.4, prob.cens = 35%, $V \sim N(0,1)$ and size = 500

	$\hat{\beta}_2$	$med(\hat{\beta}_2)$	$sd(\hat{\beta}_2)$	$\overline{sd(\hat{\beta}_2)}$	$\% \in CI$	$\widehat{MSE}$	$\widehat{E}(T)$	$\bar{\hat{\tau}}_2$	$med(\hat{\tau}_2)$	$sd(\hat{\tau}_2)$	$\overline{sd(\hat{\tau}_2)}$	$\% \in CI$	$\widehat{MSE}$
sd.U = 0													
benchmark	-0.203	-0.204	0.055	0.053	94.200	0.003	0.903	-0.409	-0.410	0.061	0.061	94.200	0.004
naive	-0.203	-0.204	0.055	0.053	94.200	0.003	0.903	-0.409	-0.410	0.061	0.061	94.200	0.004
reg.calib	-0.203	-0.204	0.055	0.053	94.200	0.003	0.903	-0.409	-0.410	0.061	0.061	94.200	0.004
corr	-0.203	-0.204	0.055	0.053	93.400	0.003	0.903	-0.409	-0.410	0.061	0.060	94.000	0.004
sd.U = 0.1													
benchmark	-0.203	-0.204	0.054	0.053	94.600	0.003	0.904	-0.405	-0.402	0.064	0.061	94.800	0.004
naive	-0.201	-0.202	0.054	0.053	94.200	0.003	0.904	-0.405	-0.401	0.064	0.061	95.000	0.004
reg.calib	-0.203	-0.204	0.054	0.054	94.600	0.003	0.904	-0.405	-0.401	0.064	0.061	95.000	0.004
corr	-0.203	-0.205	0.055	0.053	94.000	0.003	0.904	-0.405	-0.401	0.064	0.060	93.800	0.004
sd.U = 0.4													
benchmark	-0.198	-0.201	0.054	0.053	94.400	0.003	0.904	-0.406	-0.405	0.062	0.061	95.000	0.004
naive	-0.170	-0.169	0.051	0.050	89.400	0.003	0.905	-0.400	-0.401	0.062	0.061	93.800	0.004
reg.calib	-0.197	-0.195	0.059	0.058	93.400	0.003	0.905	-0.400	-0.401	0.062	0.061	93.800	0.004
corr	-0.198	-0.197	0.060	0.057	93.600	0.004	0.904	-0.406	-0.406	0.063	0.061	94.000	0.004
sd.U = 0.8													
benchmark	-0.203	-0.203	0.052	0.053	95.600	0.003	0.904	-0.408	-0.405	0.059	0.061	94.800	0.004
naive	-0.123	-0.122	0.042	0.042	53.200	0.008	0.905	-0.394	-0.393	0.059	0.061	95.800	0.003
reg.calib	-0.202	-0.201	0.069	0.069	95.400	0.005	0.905	-0.394	-0.393	0.059	0.061	95.800	0.003
corr	-0.208	-0.204	0.077	0.074	95.600	0.006	0.903	-0.411	-0.408	0.062	0.064	95.000	0.004

Table C.30.: Results for node 3 with beta.1.true = 0.6, beta.2.true = -0.2 , tau.1.true = 0.5, tau.2.true = -0.4, prob.cens = 35%, $V \sim N(0,1)$ and size = 500

	%#mob	#mob	not #mob	#NA
sd.U = 0				
benchmark	100	500	0	0
naive	100	500	0	0
reg.calib	100	500	0	0
corr	100	500	0	0
sd.U = 0.1				
benchmark	100	500	0	0
naive	100	500	0	0
reg.calib	100	500	0	0
corr	100	500	0	0
sd.U = 0.4				
benchmark	100	500	0	0
naive	100	500	0	0
reg.calib	100	500	0	0
corr	100	500	0	0
sd.U = 0.8				
benchmark	100	500	0	0
naive	100	500	0	0
reg.calib	100	500	0	0
corr	100	500	0	0

Table C.31.: Detection of the true structural change with `beta.1.true` = 0.6, `beta.2.true` = -0.2 , `tau.1.true` = 0.5, `tau.2.true` = -0.4, `prob.cens` = 35%, $V \sim N(0,1)$ and `size` = 1000

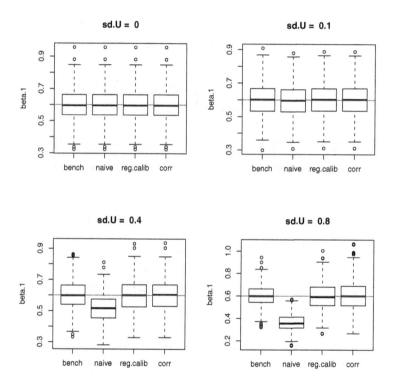

Figure C.51.: Boxplot for β_1 with beta.1.true $= 0.6$, beta.2.true $= -0.2$, tau.1.true $= 0.5$, tau.2.true $= -0.4$, prob.cens $= 35\%$, $V \sim N(0,1)$, size $= 1000$

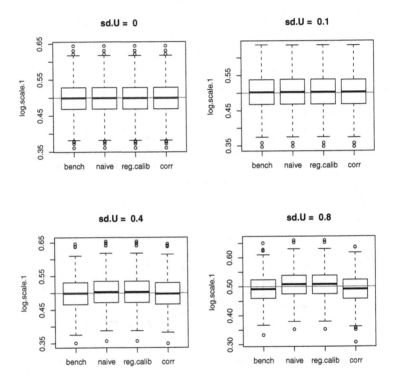

Figure C.52.: Boxplot for τ_1 with beta.1.true $= 0.6$, beta.2.true $= -0.2$, tau.1.true $= 0.5$, tau.2.true $= -0.4$, prob.cens $= 35\%$, $V \sim N(0,1)$, size $= 1000$

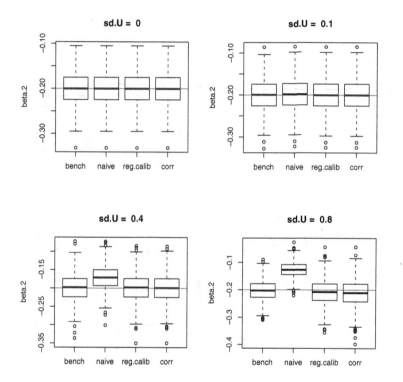

Figure C.53.: Boxplot for β_2 with beta.1.true = 0.6, beta.2.true = -0.2 , tau.1.true = 0.5, tau.2.true = -0.4, prob.cens = 35%, $V \sim N(0,1)$, size = 1000

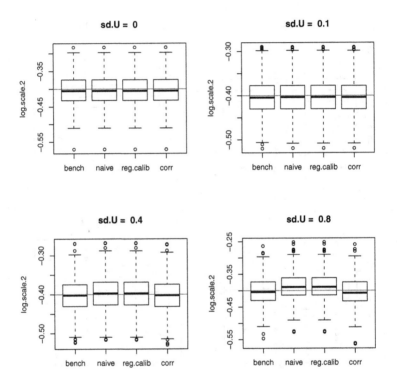

Figure C.54.: Boxplot for τ_2 with beta.1.true $= 0.6$, beta.2.true $= -0.2$, tau.1.true $= 0.5$, tau.2.true $= -0.4$, prob.cens $= 35\%$, $V \sim N(0,1)$, size $= 1000$

	$\hat{\bar{\beta}}_1$	$med(\hat{\beta}_1)$	$sd(\hat{\beta}_1)$	$\overline{sd(\hat{\beta}_1)}$	$\% \in CI$	$\widehat{MSE}$	$\widehat{E(T)}$	$\bar{\hat{\tau}}_1$	$med(\hat{\tau}_1)$	$sd(\hat{\tau}_1)$	$\overline{sd(\hat{\tau}_1)}$	$\% \in CI$	$\widehat{MSE}$
sd.U = 0													
benchmark	0.599	0.597	0.098	0.096	94.600	0.010	1.486	0.498	0.499	0.048	0.047	92.000	0.002
naive	0.599	0.597	0.098	0.096	94.600	0.010	1.486	0.498	0.499	0.048	0.047	92.000	0.002
reg.calib	0.599	0.597	0.098	0.096	94.600	0.010	1.486	0.498	0.499	0.048	0.047	92.000	0.002
corr	0.599	0.597	0.098	0.096	94.400	0.010	1.486	0.498	0.499	0.048	0.047	91.600	0.002
sd.U = 0.1													
benchmark	0.601	0.602	0.096	0.097	95.400	0.009	1.494	0.501	0.502	0.050	0.048	94.200	0.003
naive	0.595	0.596	0.095	0.097	95.200	0.009	1.495	0.501	0.502	0.050	0.048	94.200	0.003
reg.calib	0.601	0.603	0.096	0.098	95.600	0.009	1.495	0.501	0.502	0.050	0.048	94.200	0.003
corr	0.602	0.603	0.096	0.097	95.600	0.009	1.494	0.501	0.502	0.050	0.047	94.400	0.003
sd.U = 0.4													
benchmark	0.601	0.599	0.095	0.096	95.600	0.009	1.491	0.499	0.499	0.049	0.047	94.000	0.002
naive	0.517	0.517	0.090	0.089	82.000	0.015	1.501	0.505	0.503	0.049	0.047	93.800	0.002
reg.calib	0.600	0.601	0.104	0.104	95.400	0.011	1.501	0.505	0.503	0.049	0.047	93.800	0.002
corr	0.603	0.604	0.105	0.105	95.600	0.011	1.491	0.499	0.498	0.049	0.048	93.400	0.002
sd.U = 0.8													
benchmark	0.605	0.600	0.096	0.096	95.800	0.009	1.476	0.492	0.492	0.048	0.047	94.200	0.002
naive	0.363	0.357	0.072	0.075	11.600	0.061	1.506	0.507	0.508	0.048	0.048	93.800	0.002
reg.calib	0.596	0.592	0.121	0.123	96.600	0.015	1.507	0.507	0.508	0.048	0.048	93.800	0.002
corr	0.608	0.601	0.130	0.133	96.000	0.017	1.476	0.491	0.491	0.050	0.049	93.600	0.003

Table C.32.: Results for node 2 with beta.1.true = 0.6, beta.2.true = -0.2, tau.1.true = 0.5, tau.2.true = -0.4, prob.cens = 35%, $V \sim N(0,1)$ and size = 1000

	$\hat{\bar{\beta}}_2$	$med(\hat{\beta}_2)$	$sd(\hat{\beta}_2)$	$\widehat{sd(\hat{\beta}_2)}$	$\% \in CI$	$\widehat{MSE}$	$\mathbb{E}(T)$	$\hat{\bar{\tau}}_2$	$med(\hat{\tau}_2)$	$sd(\hat{\tau}_2)$	$\widehat{sd(\hat{\tau}_2)}$	$\% \in CI$	$\widehat{MSE}$
sd.U = 0													
benchmark	-0.200	-0.200	0.037	0.037	94.200	0.001	0.904	-0.404	-0.405	0.042	0.043	94.800	0.002
naive	-0.200	-0.200	0.037	0.037	94.200	0.001	0.904	-0.404	-0.405	0.042	0.043	94.800	0.002
reg.calib	-0.200	-0.200	0.037	0.037	94.200	0.001	0.904	-0.404	-0.405	0.042	0.043	94.800	0.002
corr	-0.200	-0.200	0.037	0.037	94.400	0.001	0.904	-0.404	-0.405	0.042	0.043	94.600	0.002
sd.U = 0.1													
benchmark	-0.200	-0.199	0.038	0.037	93.800	0.001	0.904	-0.403	-0.404	0.042	0.043	95.200	0.002
naive	-0.198	-0.198	0.038	0.037	93.200	0.001	0.904	-0.403	-0.403	0.042	0.043	95.000	0.002
reg.calib	-0.200	-0.200	0.039	0.038	93.400	0.001	0.904	-0.403	-0.403	0.042	0.043	95.000	0.002
corr	-0.200	-0.200	0.039	0.038	93.200	0.001	0.904	-0.403	-0.404	0.042	0.043	95.000	0.002
sd.U = 0.4													
benchmark	-0.199	-0.198	0.037	0.038	95.600	0.001	0.903	-0.403	-0.402	0.043	0.043	94.800	0.002
naive	-0.172	-0.171	0.034	0.035	88.800	0.002	0.904	-0.398	-0.398	0.043	0.043	95.000	0.002
reg.calib	-0.200	-0.198	0.039	0.041	95.200	0.002	0.904	-0.398	-0.398	0.043	0.043	95.000	0.002
corr	-0.201	-0.199	0.039	0.041	94.400	0.002	0.903	-0.403	-0.402	0.043	0.043	95.000	0.002
sd.U = 0.8													
benchmark	-0.203	-0.202	0.038	0.037	94.800	0.001	0.903	-0.402	-0.405	0.042	0.043	95.400	0.002
naive	-0.126	-0.127	0.029	0.030	27.400	0.006	0.905	-0.389	-0.389	0.042	0.043	95.400	0.002
reg.calib	-0.207	-0.207	0.047	0.049	95.400	0.002	0.905	-0.389	-0.389	0.042	0.043	95.400	0.002
corr	-0.210	-0.211	0.051	0.051	95.000	0.003	0.903	-0.405	-0.408	0.045	0.045	95.600	0.002

Table C.33.: Results for node 3 with beta.1.true = 0.6, beta.2.true = -0.2, tau.1.true = 0.5, tau.2.true = -0.4, prob.cens = 35%, $V \sim N(0,1)$ and size = 1000

C.4. Structural Changes – multi

	size = 100				size = 500				size = 1000			
	%#mob	#mob	not #mob	#NA	%#mob	#mob	not #mob	#NA	%#mob	#mob	not #mob	#NA
sd.U = 0												
benchmark	0.4	2	498	0	1.0	5	495	0	1.4	7	493	0
naive	0.4	2	498	0	1.0	5	495	0	1.4	7	493	0
reg.calib	0.4	2	498	0	1.0	5	495	0	1.4	7	493	0
corr	0.4	2	498	0	1.0	5	495	0	1.4	7	493	0
sd.U = 0.1												
benchmark	0.0	0	500	0	1.2	6	494	0	2.4	12	488	0
naive	0.0	0	500	0	1.4	7	493	0	2.0	10	490	0
reg.calib	0.0	0	500	0	1.4	7	493	0	2.0	10	490	0
corr	0.0	0	500	0	1.4	7	493	0	2.0	10	490	0
sd.U = 0.4												
benchmark	0.0	0	500	0	1.0	5	495	0	1.6	8	492	0
naive	0.0	0	500	0	1.6	8	492	0	0.8	4	496	0
reg.calib	0.0	0	500	0	1.6	8	492	0	0.8	4	496	0
corr	0.0	0	500	0	1.6	8	492	1	0.6	3	497	0
sd.U = 0.8												
benchmark	0.0	0	500	0	2.4	12	488	0	3.2	16	484	0
naive	0.0	0	500	0	0.8	4	496	0	1.6	8	492	0
reg.calib	0.0	0	500	0	0.8	4	496	0	1.6	8	492	0
corr	0.0	0	500	1	0.8	4	496	7	0.2	1	499	10

Table C.34.: Detection of the true structural changes with beta.1.true $= -0.9$, beta.2.true $= 0.2$, beta.3.true $= 1.1$, tau.1.true $= 0.5$, tau.2.true $= 0.5$, tau.3.true $= 0.5$, prob.cens $= 0\%$, $V \sim N(0,1)$ and size $= 100, 500, 1000$

	size = 100				size = 500				size = 1000			
	%#mob	#mob	not #mob	#NA	%#mob	#mob	not #mob	#NA	%#mob	#mob	not #mob	#NA
sd.U = 0												
benchmark	0.0	0	500	0	1.0	5	495	0	1.2	6	494	0
naive	0.0	0	500	0	1.0	5	495	0	1.2	6	494	0
reg.calib	0.0	0	500	0	1.0	5	495	0	1.2	6	494	0
corr	0.0	0	500	0	1.0	5	495	0	1.2	6	494	0
sd.U = 0.1												
benchmark	0.2	1	499	0	0.6	3	497	0	1.0	5	495	0
naive	0.2	1	499	0	0.6	3	497	0	1.2	6	494	0
reg.calib	0.2	1	499	0	0.6	3	497	0	1.2	6	494	0
corr	0.2	1	499	0	0.6	3	497	0	1.2	6	494	0
sd.U = 0.4												
benchmark	0.2	1	499	0	1.4	7	493	0	2.0	10	490	0
naive	0.0	0	500	0	0.6	3	497	0	1.6	8	492	0
reg.calib	0.0	0	500	0	0.6	3	497	0	1.6	8	492	0
corr	0.0	0	500	0	0.8	4	496	0	1.8	9	491	0
sd.U = 0.8												
benchmark	0.2	1	499	0	1.2	6	494	0	2.6	13	487	0
naive	0.0	0	500	0	1.2	6	494	0	1.2	6	494	0
reg.calib	0.0	0	500	0	1.2	6	494	0	1.2	6	494	0
corr	0.0	0	500	5	0.0	0	500	7	0.6	3	497	7

Table C.35.: Detection of the true structural changes with beta.1.true = −0.9, beta.2.true = 0.2, beta.3.true = 1.1, tau.1.true = 0.5, tau.2.true = 0.5, tau.3.true = 0.5, prob.cens = 35%, $V \sim N(0,1)$ and size = 100, 500, 1000

	size = 100				size = 500				size = 1000			
	%#mob	#mob	not #mob	#NA	%#mob	#mob	not #mob	#NA	%#mob	#mob	not #mob	#NA
sd.U = 0												
benchmark	0	0	500	0	0.6	3	497	0	1.2	6	494	0
naive	0	0	500	0	0.6	3	497	0	1.2	6	494	0
reg.calib	0	0	500	0	0.6	3	497	0	1.2	6	494	0
corr	0	0	500	0	0.6	3	497	0	1.2	6	494	0
sd.U = 0.1												
benchmark	0	0	500	0	0.6	3	497	0	0.8	4	496	0
naive	0	0	500	0	0.4	2	498	0	0.6	3	497	0
reg.calib	0	0	500	0	0.4	2	498	0	0.6	3	497	0
corr	0	0	500	0	0.4	2	498	0	0.6	3	497	0
sd.U = 0.4												
benchmark	0	0	500	0	0.2	1	499	0	0.6	3	497	0
naive	0	0	500	0	0.2	1	499	0	1.2	6	494	0
reg.calib	0	0	500	0	0.2	1	499	0	1.2	6	494	0
corr	0	0	500	0	0.2	1	499	1	1.4	7	493	0
sd.U = 0.8												
benchmark	0	0	500	0	0.8	4	496	0	1.4	7	493	0
naive	0	0	500	0	0.4	2	498	0	0.6	3	497	0
reg.calib	0	0	500	0	0.4	2	498	0	0.6	3	497	0
corr	0	0	500	1	0.0	0	500	15	0.4	2	498	6

Table C.36.: Detection of the true structural changes with beta.1.true = −0.9, beta.2.true = 0.2, beta.3.true = 1.1, tau.1.true = 0.5, tau.2.true = 0.5, tau.3.true = 0.5, prob.cens = 65%, $V \sim N(0,1)$ and size = 100, 500, 1000

	size = 100				size = 500				size = 1000			
	%#mob	#mob	not #mob	#NA	%#mob	#mob	not #mob	#NA	%#mob	#mob	not #mob	#NA
sd.U = 0												
benchmark	0.4	2	498	0	3.0	15	485	0	1.6	8	492	0
naive	0.4	2	498	0	3.0	15	485	0	1.6	8	492	0
reg.calib	0.4	2	498	0	3.0	15	485	0	1.6	8	492	0
corr	0.4	2	498	0	3.0	15	485	0	1.4	7	493	1
sd.U = 0.1												
benchmark	0.0	0	500	0	3.8	19	481	0	3.2	16	484	0
naive	0.0	0	500	0	3.6	18	482	0	3.4	17	483	0
reg.calib	0.0	0	500	0	3.6	18	482	0	3.4	17	483	0
corr	0.0	0	500	1	3.6	18	482	0	3.4	17	483	0
sd.U = 0.4												
benchmark	0.0	0	500	0	1.0	5	495	0	1.4	7	493	0
naive	0.0	0	500	0	1.2	6	494	0	2.8	14	486	0
reg.calib	0.0	0	500	0	1.2	6	494	0	2.8	14	486	0
corr	0.0	0	500	1	1.0	5	495	1	2.8	14	486	0
sd.U = 0.8												
benchmark	0.2	1	499	0	2.2	11	489	0	2.4	12	488	0
naive	0.2	1	499	0	2.8	14	486	0	2.8	14	486	0
reg.calib	0.2	1	499	0	2.8	14	486	0	2.8	14	486	0
corr	0.0	0	500	9	1.8	9	491	13	0.8	4	496	10

Table C.37.: Detection of the true structural changes with beta.1.true = 0.4, beta.2.true = 0.4, beta.3.true = 0.4, tau.1.true = -1, tau.2.true = 0.1, tau.3.true = 0.9, prob.cens = 0%, $V \sim N(0,1)$ and size = 100, 500, 1000

	size = 100				size = 500				size = 1000			
	%#mob	#mob	not #mob	#NA	%#mob	#mob	not #mob	#NA	%#mob	#mob	not #mob	#NA
sd.U = 0												
benchmark	0.2	1	499	0	1.4	7	493	0	2.8	14	486	0
naive	0.2	1	499	0	1.4	7	493	0	2.8	14	486	0
reg.calib	0.2	1	499	0	1.4	7	493	0	2.8	14	486	0
corr	0.2	1	499	0	1.4	7	493	10	2.8	14	486	4
sd.U = 0.1												
benchmark	1.2	6	494	0	2.0	10	490	0	1.2	6	494	0
naive	1.2	6	494	0	1.8	9	491	0	1.2	6	494	0
reg.calib	1.2	6	494	0	1.8	9	491	0	1.2	6	494	0
corr	1.2	6	494	1	1.6	8	492	6	1.2	6	494	4
sd.U = 0.4												
benchmark	1.0	5	495	0	1.2	6	494	0	2.0	10	490	0
naive	0.8	4	496	0	1.0	5	495	0	2.6	13	487	0
reg.calib	0.8	4	496	0	1.0	5	495	0	2.6	13	487	0
corr	0.8	4	496	10	1.4	7	493	2	2.2	11	489	13
sd.U = 0.8												
benchmark	0.2	1	499	0	3.6	18	482	0	2.0	10	490	0
naive	0.6	3	497	0	2.4	12	488	0	2.2	11	489	0
reg.calib	0.6	3	497	0	2.4	12	488	0	2.2	11	489	0
corr	0.0	0	500	246	1.0	5	495	19	0.6	3	497	16

Table C.38.: Detection of the true structural changes with beta.1.true = 0.4, beta.2.true = 0.4, beta.3.true = 0.4, tau.1.true = -1, tau.2.true = 0.1, tau.3.true = 0.9, prob.cens = 35%, $V \sim N(0,1)$ and size = 100, 500, 1000

	size = 100				size = 500				size = 1000			
	%#mob	#mob	not #mob	#NA	%#mob	#mob	not #mob	#NA	%#mob	#mob	not #mob	#NA
sd.U = 0												
benchmark	0.8	4	496	0	2.8	14	486	3	2.2	11	489	0
naive	0.8	4	496	0	2.8	14	486	3	2.2	11	489	0
reg.calib	0.8	4	496	0	2.8	14	486	3	2.2	11	489	0
corr	0.8	4	496	3	2.8	14	486	9	2.2	11	489	6
sd.U = 0.1												
benchmark	0.6	3	497	0	1.0	5	495	1	1.4	7	493	0
naive	0.6	3	497	0	2.0	10	490	0	1.4	7	493	0
reg.calib	0.6	3	497	0	2.0	10	490	0	1.4	7	493	0
corr	0.6	3	497	1	2.0	10	490	3	1.4	7	493	5
sd.U = 0.4												
benchmark	1.2	6	494	0	1.2	6	494	0	2.0	10	490	0
naive	1.0	5	495	0	2.4	12	488	1	2.8	14	486	0
reg.calib	1.0	5	495	0	2.4	12	488	1	2.8	14	486	0
corr	0.8	4	496	3	2.2	11	489	5	1.8	9	491	7
sd.U = 0.8												
benchmark	0.2	1	499	0	0.8	4	496	0	2.0	10	490	1
naive	0.0	0	500	0	2.0	10	490	0	2.2	11	489	2
reg.calib	0.0	0	500	0	2.0	10	490	0	2.2	11	489	2
corr	0.0	0	500	6	0.6	3	497	13	0.6	3	497	19

Table C.39.: Detection of the true structural changes with beta.1.true = 0.4, beta.2.true = 0.4, beta.3.true = 0.4, tau.1.true = -1, tau.2.true = 0.1, tau.3.true = 0.9, prob.cens = 65%, $V \sim N(0,1)$ and size = 100, 500, 1000

	size = 100				size = 500				size = 1000			
	%#mob	#mob	not #mob	#NA	%#mob	#mob	not #mob	#NA	%#mob	#mob	not #mob	#NA
sd.U = 0												
benchmark	0.0	0	500	0	2.8	14	486	0	2.0	10	490	0
naive	0.0	0	500	0	2.8	14	486	0	2.0	10	490	0
reg.calib	0.0	0	500	0	2.8	14	486	0	2.0	10	490	0
corr	0.0	0	500	1	2.8	14	486	0	2.0	10	490	0
sd.U = 0.1												
benchmark	0.2	1	499	0	2.2	11	489	0	2.8	14	486	0
naive	0.2	1	499	0	2.4	12	488	0	2.4	12	488	0
reg.calib	0.2	1	499	0	2.4	12	488	0	2.4	12	488	0
corr	0.2	1	499	0	2.4	12	488	0	2.4	12	488	0
sd.U = 0.4												
benchmark	0.2	1	499	0	2.0	10	490	0	3.6	18	482	0
naive	0.2	1	499	0	1.6	8	492	0	2.6	13	487	0
reg.calib	0.2	1	499	0	1.6	8	492	0	2.6	13	487	0
corr	0.2	1	499	6	1.2	6	494	11	2.8	14	486	18
sd.U = 0.8												
benchmark	0.0	0	500	0	2.4	12	488	0	2.8	14	486	0
naive	0.6	3	497	0	3.0	15	485	0	2.4	12	488	0
reg.calib	0.6	3	497	0	3.0	15	485	0	2.4	12	488	0
corr	0.0	0	500	4	0.2	1	499	24	0.2	1	499	16

Table C.40.: Detection of the true structural changes with $beta.1.true = -0.9$, $beta.2.true = 0.2$, $beta.3.true = 1.1$, $tau.1.true = -1$, $tau.2.true = 0.1$, $tau.3.true = 0.9$, $prob.cens = 0\%$, $V \sim N(0,1)$ and $size = 100, 500, 1000$

	size = 100				size = 500				size = 1000			
	%#mob	#mob	not #mob	#NA	%#mob	#mob	not #mob	#NA	%#mob	#mob	not #mob	#NA
sd.U = 0												
benchmark	0.4	2	498	0	1.4	7	493	0	1.6	8	492	0
naive	0.4	2	498	0	1.4	7	493	0	1.6	8	492	0
reg.calib	0.4	2	498	0	1.4	7	493	0	1.6	8	492	0
corr	0.4	2	498	2	1.4	7	493	2	1.6	8	492	2
sd.U = 0.1												
benchmark	0.6	3	497	0	1.2	6	494	0	2.2	11	489	0
naive	0.2	1	499	0	1.0	5	495	0	1.8	9	491	0
reg.calib	0.2	1	499	0	1.0	5	495	0	1.8	9	491	0
corr	0.2	1	499	0	1.0	5	495	4	1.8	9	491	4
sd.U = 0.4												
benchmark	0.2	1	499	0	2.0	10	490	0	1.8	9	491	0
naive	0.2	1	499	0	1.6	8	492	0	2.4	12	488	0
reg.calib	0.2	1	499	0	1.6	8	492	0	2.4	12	488	0
corr	0.2	1	499	6	1.8	9	491	12	2.4	12	488	13
sd.U = 0.8												
benchmark	0.2	1	499	0	1.0	5	495	0	2.4	12	488	0
naive	0.2	1	499	0	0.8	4	496	0	2.6	13	487	0
reg.calib	0.2	1	499	0	0.8	4	496	0	2.6	13	487	0
corr	0.0	0	500	14	0.0	0	500	12	0.0	0	500	22

Table C.41.: Detection of the true structural changes with beta.1.true = -0.9, beta.2.true = 0.2 , beta.3.true = 1.1, tau.1.true = -1, tau.2.true = 0.1, tau.3.true = 0.9, prob.cens = 35%, $V \sim N(0,1)$ and size = 100, 500, 1000

	size = 100				size = 500				size = 1000			
	%#mob	#mob	not #mob	#NA	%#mob	#mob	not #mob	#NA	%#mob	#mob	not #mob	#NA
sd.U = 0												
benchmark	0.2	1	499	0	2.2	11	489	0	2.4	12	488	0
naive	0.2	1	499	0	2.2	11	489	0	2.4	12	488	0
reg.calib	0.2	1	499	0	2.2	11	489	0	2.4	12	488	0
corr	0.2	1	499	5	2.2	11	489	10	2.4	12	488	20
sd.U = 0.1												
benchmark	1.2	6	494	0	1.6	8	492	0	1.4	7	493	0
naive	1.0	5	495	0	1.6	8	492	0	1.2	6	494	0
reg.calib	1.0	5	495	0	1.6	8	492	0	1.2	6	494	0
corr	1.2	6	494	2	1.4	7	493	15	1.2	6	494	12
sd.U = 0.4												
benchmark	0.8	4	496	0	2.0	10	490	0	2.8	14	486	0
naive	1.0	5	495	0	1.8	9	491	1	2.8	14	486	1
reg.calib	1.0	5	495	0	1.8	9	491	1	2.8	14	486	1
corr	0.0	0	500	14	1.6	8	492	17	2.6	13	487	25
sd.U = 0.8												
benchmark	0.2	1	499	0	1.8	9	491	0	1.8	9	491	0
naive	0.6	3	497	0	1.2	6	494	1	1.4	7	493	0
reg.calib	0.6	3	497	0	1.2	6	494	1	1.4	7	493	0
corr	0.0	0	500	17	0.0	0	500	12	0.0	0	500	15

Table C.42.: Detection of the true structural changes with beta.1.true = -0.9, beta.2.true = 0.2, beta.3.true = 1.1, tau.1.true = -1, tau.2.true = 0.1, tau.3.true = 0.9, prob.cens = 65%, $V \sim N(0,1)$ and size = 100, 500, 1000

C.4.1. Summary of Parameter Estimation

For sd.U = 0.4 with beta.1.true = -0.9, beta.2.true = 0.2 , beta.3.true = 1.1, tau.1.true = -1, tau.2.true = 0.1, tau.3.true = 0.9, prob.cens = 0% and $V \sim N(0,1)$.

Benchmark Estimation

```
> summary(mob.results.benchmark)
$'2'


Call:
survreg(formula = y ~ ., data = mydata, weights = weights)
             Value Std. Error    z        p
(Intercept) -0.0316    0.0187  -1.69  9.11e-02
V           -0.8843    0.0187 -47.40  0.00e+00 # beta.1.true = -0.9
Log(scale)  -0.9629    0.0352 -27.38 4.22e-165 # tau.1.true = -1

Scale= 0.382


Weibull distribution
Loglik(model)= -195.8   Loglik(intercept only)= -581.8
        Chisq= 771.95 on 1 degrees of freedom, p= 0
Number of Newton-Raphson Iterations: 6
n= 466



$'4'


Call:
survreg(formula = y ~ ., data = mydata, weights = weights)
             Value Std. Error    z       p
(Intercept) 0.0333    0.0721 0.462 0.64440
V           0.1804     0.0624 2.894 0.00381 # beta.2.true = 0.2
Log(scale)  0.0812     0.0482 1.686 0.09174 # tau.2.true = 0.1

Scale= 1.08
```

```
Weibull distribution
Loglik(model)= -268   Loglik(intercept only)= -272
      Chisq= 8.06 on 1 degrees of freedom, p= 0.0045
Number of Newton-Raphson Iterations: 5
n= 252
```

```
$'5'
```

```
Call:
survreg(formula = y ~ ., data = mydata, weights = weights)
            Value Std. Error    z       p
(Intercept) 0.0605    0.1479 0.409 6.83e-01
V           0.9853    0.1465 6.725 1.75e-11 # beta.3.true = 1.1
Log(scale)  0.8576    0.0466 18.399 1.34e-75 # tau.3.true = 0.9
```

```
Scale= 2.36
```

```
Weibull distribution
Loglik(model)= -326   Loglik(intercept only)= -346.3
      Chisq= 40.63 on 1 degrees of freedom, p= 1.8e-10
Number of Newton-Raphson Iterations: 6
n= 282
```

Naive Estimation

```
> summary(mob.results.naive)
$'2'
```

```
Call:
survreg(formula = y ~ ., data = mydata, weights = weights)
              Value Std. Error    z        p
(Intercept) 0.00231    0.0246  0.094 9.25e-01
W          -0.75601    0.0220 -34.308 6.06e-258 # beta.1.true = -0.9
Log(scale) -0.69624    0.0336 -20.742 1.45e-95 # tau.1.true = -1
```

Scale= 0.498

Weibull distribution
Loglik(model)= -306.1   Loglik(intercept only)= -581.8
        Chisq= 551.41 on 1 degrees of freedom, p= 0
Number of Newton-Raphson Iterations: 6
n= 466

$'4'

Call:
survreg(formula = y ~ ., data = mydata, weights = weights)
            Value Std. Error   z   p
(Intercept) 0.0381   0.0726 0.525 0.59993
W   0.1529   0.0579 2.641 0.00827 # beta.2.true = 0.2
Log(scale) 0.0865   0.0480 1.803 0.07134 # tau.2.true = 0.1

Scale= 1.09

Weibull distribution
Loglik(model)= -268.6   Loglik(intercept only)= -272
        Chisq= 6.79 on 1 degrees of freedom, p= 0.0092
Number of Newton-Raphson Iterations: 5
n= 252

$'5'

Call:
survreg(formula = y ~ ., data = mydata, weights = weights)
            Value Std. Error   z   p
(Intercept) 0.106   0.1513 0.703 4.82e-01
W   0.797   0.1443 5.527 3.26e-08 # beta.3.true = 1.1
Log(scale) 0.880   0.0466 18.897 1.21e-79 # tau.3.true = 0.9

```
Scale= 2.41


Weibull distribution
Loglik(model)= -331.9   Loglik(intercept only)= -346.3
        Chisq= 28.69 on 1 degrees of freedom, p= 8.5e-08
Number of Newton-Raphson Iterations: 6
n= 282
```

Regression Calibration

```
> summary(mob.results.reg.calib)
$'2'


Call:
survreg(formula = y ~ ., data = mydata, weights = weights)
               Value Std. Error     z        p
(Intercept) -0.00597     0.0246  -0.243  8.08e-01
W.reg.calib -0.88164     0.0257 -34.308  6.06e-258 # beta.1.true = -0.9
Log(scale)  -0.69624     0.0336 -20.742  1.45e-95 # tau.1.true = -1


Scale= 0.498


Weibull distribution
Loglik(model)= -306.1   Loglik(intercept only)= -581.8
        Chisq= 551.41 on 1 degrees of freedom, p= 0
Number of Newton-Raphson Iterations: 6
n= 466



$'4'


Call:
survreg(formula = y ~ ., data = mydata, weights = weights)
              Value Std. Error     z       p
(Intercept) 0.0397     0.0726  0.547  0.58414
```

```
W.reg.calib 0.1784     0.0675 2.641 0.00827 # beta.2.true = 0.2
Log(scale)  0.0865     0.0480 1.803 0.07134 # tau.2.true = 0.1


Scale= 1.09


Weibull distribution
Loglik(model)= -268.6   Loglik(intercept only)= -272
        Chisq= 6.79 on 1 degrees of freedom, p= 0.0092
Number of Newton-Raphson Iterations: 5
n= 252



$'5'


Call:
survreg(formula = y ~ ., data = mydata, weights = weights)
            Value Std. Error     z        p
(Intercept) 0.115     0.1513  0.761 4.47e-01
W.reg.calib 0.930     0.1682  5.527 3.26e-08 # beta.3.true = 1.1
Log(scale)  0.880     0.0466 18.897 1.21e-79 # tau.3.true = 0.9


Scale= 2.41


Weibull distribution
Loglik(model)= -331.9   Loglik(intercept only)= -346.3
        Chisq= 28.69 on 1 degrees of freedom, p= 8.5e-08
Number of Newton-Raphson Iterations: 6
n= 282
```

Corrected Estimation

```
> summary(mob.results.corr)
$'2'


Call:
optim(model.par.naive, minus.log.lik.weibull, method = "Nelder-Mead",
```

```
    hessian = TRUE)
             Value Std. Error    z        p
Intercept  -0.0743   0.0276  -2.69  7.11e-03
W          -0.8754   0.0285 -30.72  3.35e-207 # beta.1.true = -0.9
Log(scale) -0.9860   0.1137  -8.67  4.21e-18 # tau.1.true = -1


Scale= 0.373


Weibull distribution
Loglik(model)= -174.9   Loglik(intercept only)= -581.8
        Chisq= 813.78 on 1 degrees of freedom, p= 0
Number of Newton-Raphson Iterations: 88
n= 466



$'4'


Call:
optim(model.par.naive, minus.log.lik.weibull, method = "Nelder-Mead",
    hessian = TRUE)
             Value Std. Error    z        p
Intercept   0.0384   0.0729 0.527  0.59826
W           0.1726   0.0619 2.790  0.00527 # beta.2.true = 0.2
Log(scale)  0.0840   0.0492 1.708  0.08772 # tau.2.true = 0.1


Scale= 1.09


Weibull distribution
Loglik(model)= -268.2   Loglik(intercept only)= -272
        Chisq= 7.69 on 1 degrees of freedom, p= 0.0056
Number of Newton-Raphson Iterations: 48
n= 252



$'5'
```

```
Call:
optim(model.par.naive, minus.log.lik.weibull, method = "Nelder-Mead",
    hessian = TRUE)
              Value Std. Error      z        p
Intercept   0.0933      0.1519  0.614 5.39e-01
W           0.9498      0.1696  5.600 2.14e-08 # beta.3.true = 1.1
Log(scale)  0.8677      0.0453 19.164 7.33e-82 # tau.3.true = 0.9

Scale= 2.38

Weibull distribution
Loglik(model)= -329   Loglik(intercept only)= -346.3
        Chisq= 34.64 on 1 degrees of freedom, p= 4e-09
Number of Newton-Raphson Iterations: 62
n= 282
```

C.5. One Global Model Fit vs. MOB

C.5.1. beta.1.true $= \mathbf{0.6}$, beta.2.true $= \mathbf{-0.2}$, tau.1.true $= \mathbf{0.5}$, tau.2.true $= \mathbf{-0.4}$, prob.cens $= \mathbf{0\%}$ and $V \sim N(0, 1)$

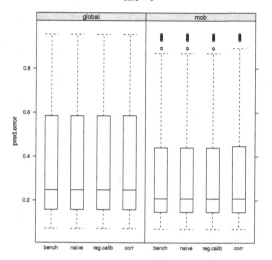

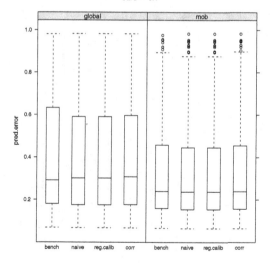

Figure C.55.: Boxplot for beta.1.true = 0.6, beta.2.true = -0.2 , tau.1.true = 0.5, tau.2.true = -0.4, prob.cens = 0% and $V \sim N(0,1)$, size = 100, sd.U = 0 and sd.U = 0.1

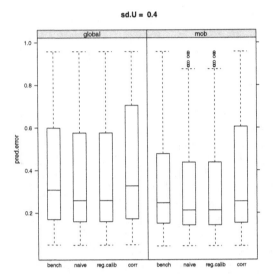

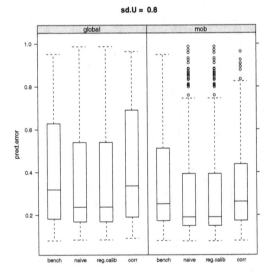

Figure C.56.: Boxplot for beta.1.true = 0.6, beta.2.true = -0.2 , tau.1.true = 0.5, tau.2.true = -0.4, prob.cens = 0% and $V \sim N(0,1)$, size = 100, sd.U = 0.4 and sd.U = 0.8

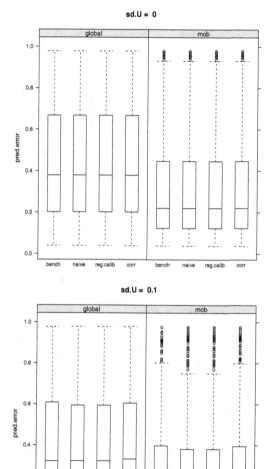

Figure C.57.: Boxplot for beta.1.true $= 0.6$, beta.2.true $= -0.2$, tau.1.true $= 0.5$, tau.2.true $= -0.4$, prob.cens $= 0\%$ and $V \sim N(0,1)$, size $= 500$, sd.U $= 0$ and sd.U $= 0.1$

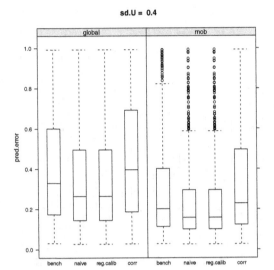

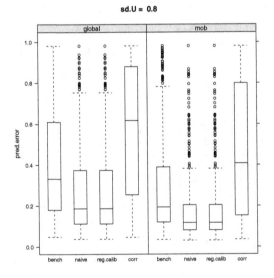

Figure C.58.: Boxplot for beta.1.true = 0.6, beta.2.true = -0.2 , tau.1.true = 0.5, tau.2.true = -0.4, prob.cens = 0% and $V \sim N(0,1)$, size = 500, sd.U = 0.4 and sd.U = 0.8

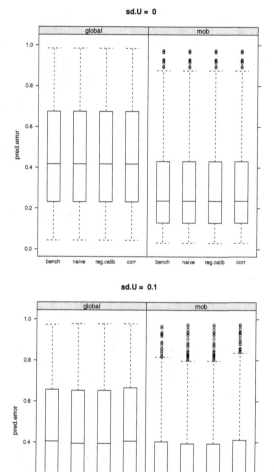

Figure C.59.: Boxplot for beta.1.true = 0.6, beta.2.true = -0.2 , tau.1.true = 0.5, tau.2.true = -0.4, prob.cens = 0% and $V \sim N(0,1)$, size = 1000, sd.U = 0 and sd.U = 0.1

sd.U = 0.4

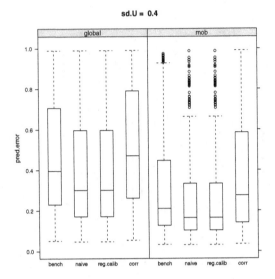

sd.U = 0.8

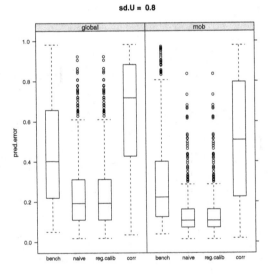

Figure C.60.: Boxplot for beta.1.true = 0.6, beta.2.true = -0.2 , tau.1.true = 0.5, tau.2.true = -0.4, prob.cens = 0% and $V \sim N(0,1)$, size = 1000, sd.U = 0.4 and sd.U = 0.8

	global		mob		
	`ierror`	`CI`	`ierror`	`CI`	`#NA`
sd.U = 0					
benchmark	0.247	[0.089,0.941]	0.209	[0.090,0.935]	276
naive	0.247	[0.089,0.941]	0.209	[0.090,0.935]	276
reg.calib	0.247	[0.089,0.941]	0.209	[0.090,0.935]	276
corr	0.247	[0.089,0.941]	0.209	[0.090,0.935]	278
sd.U = 0.1					
benchmark	0.292	[0.096,0.944]	0.239	[0.083,0.920]	278
naive	0.302	[0.093,0.943]	0.237	[0.081,0.926]	277
reg.calib	0.302	[0.093,0.943]	0.237	[0.081,0.926]	277
corr	0.309	[0.093,0.945]	0.239	[0.081,0.928]	277
sd.U = 0.4					
benchmark	0.309	[0.074,0.926]	0.247	[0.074,0.915]	271
naive	0.259	[0.075,0.904]	0.213	[0.074,0.890]	281
reg.calib	0.259	[0.075,0.904]	0.213	[0.074,0.890]	281
corr	0.328	[0.075,0.923]	0.255	[0.074,0.910]	282
sd.U = 0.8					
benchmark	0.320	[0.091,0.915]	0.252	[0.084,0.895]	307
naive	0.238	[0.098,0.925]	0.190	[0.089,0.924]	311
reg.calib	0.238	[0.098,0.925]	0.190	[0.089,0.924]	311
corr	0.336	[0.117,0.918]	0.263	[0.103,0.909]	419

Table C.43.: Prediction error with 95% confidence interval with `beta.1.true` = 0.6, `beta.2.true` = -0.2 , `tau.1.true` = 0.5, `tau.2.true` = -0.4, `prob.cens` = 0%, $V \sim N(0,1)$ and `size` = 100

	global		mob		
	ierror	CI	ierror	CI	#NA
sd.U = 0					
benchmark	0.379	[0.070,0.951]	0.221	[0.053,0.911]	4
naive	0.379	[0.070,0.951]	0.221	[0.053,0.911]	4
reg.calib	0.379	[0.070,0.951]	0.221	[0.053,0.911]	4
corr	0.379	[0.070,0.951]	0.221	[0.053,0.911]	4
sd.U = 0.1					
benchmark	0.322	[0.076,0.939]	0.193	[0.062,0.908]	1
naive	0.323	[0.075,0.946]	0.194	[0.061,0.914]	1
reg.calib	0.323	[0.075,0.946]	0.194	[0.061,0.914]	1
corr	0.332	[0.075,0.949]	0.198	[0.062,0.919]	1
sd.U = 0.4					
benchmark	0.330	[0.071,0.950]	0.201	[0.057,0.914]	1
naive	0.265	[0.065,0.926]	0.157	[0.054,0.828]	1
reg.calib	0.265	[0.065,0.926]	0.157	[0.054,0.828]	1
corr	0.396	[0.072,0.955]	0.228	[0.058,0.933]	1
sd.U = 0.8					
benchmark	0.332	[0.074,0.950]	0.194	[0.059,0.932]	1
naive	0.187	[0.062,0.840]	0.117	[0.049,0.701]	4
reg.calib	0.187	[0.062,0.840]	0.117	[0.049,0.701]	4
corr	0.618	[0.091,0.961]	0.408	[0.067,0.955]	12

Table C.44.: Prediction error with 95% confidence interval with beta.1.true = 0.6, beta.2.true = -0.2 , tau.1.true = 0.5, tau.2.true = -0.4, prob.cens = 0%, $V \sim N(0,1)$ and size = 500

	global		mob		
	`ierror`	`CI`	`ierror`	`CI`	`#NA`
sd.U = 0					
benchmark	0.417	[0.088,0.945]	0.236	[0.061,0.875]	0
naive	0.417	[0.088,0.945]	0.236	[0.061,0.875]	0
reg.calib	0.417	[0.088,0.945]	0.236	[0.061,0.875]	0
corr	0.417	[0.088,0.945]	0.236	[0.061,0.875]	0
sd.U = 0.1					
benchmark	0.405	[0.089,0.946]	0.216	[0.059,0.857]	0
naive	0.394	[0.084,0.946]	0.212	[0.056,0.847]	0
reg.calib	0.394	[0.084,0.946]	0.212	[0.056,0.847]	0
corr	0.405	[0.086,0.948]	0.220	[0.057,0.858]	0
sd.U = 0.4					
benchmark	0.396	[0.093,0.957]	0.210	[0.062,0.938]	0
naive	0.302	[0.072,0.934]	0.165	[0.051,0.842]	0
reg.calib	0.302	[0.072,0.934]	0.165	[0.051,0.842]	0
corr	0.471	[0.097,0.968]	0.276	[0.063,0.952]	0
sd.U = 0.8					
benchmark	0.402	[0.083,0.946]	0.222	[0.056,0.895]	0
naive	0.192	[0.054,0.761]	0.107	[0.041,0.513]	0
reg.calib	0.192	[0.054,0.761]	0.107	[0.041,0.513]	0
corr	0.717	[0.096,0.968]	0.508	[0.069,0.967]	1

Table C.45.: Prediction error with 95% confidence interval with `beta.1.true` = 0.6, `beta.2.true` = -0.2 , `tau.1.true` = 0.5, `tau.2.true` = -0.4, `prob.cens` = 0%, $V \sim N(0,1)$ and `size` = 1000

Bibliography

Andrews, D. W. K. (1993). Tests for Parameter Instability and Structural Change With Unknown Change Point. *Econometrica 61*(4), 821–856.

Andrews, D. W. K. and W. Ploberger (1994). Optimal Tests When a Nuisance Parameter Is Present Only under the Alternative. *Econometrica 62*(6), 1383–1414.

Augustin, T. (2004). An Exact Corrected Log-Likelihood Function for Cox's Proportional Hazards Model under Measurement Error and Some Extensions. *Scandinavian Journal of Statistics 31*, 43–50.

Augustin, T. and R. Schwarz (2002). Cox's Proportional Hazards Model under Covariate Measurement Error – a Review and Comparison of Methods. In: S. Van Huffel and P. Lemmerling (eds.). Total least squares and errors-in-variables modeling: analysis, algorithms and applications. Kluwer, Dordrecht, pp.175–184.

Bender, R., T. Augustin, and M. Blettner (2005). Generating Survival Times to Simulate Cox Proportional Hazards Models. *Statistics in Medicine 24*, 1713–1723.

Breiman, L. (1996). Bagging Predictors. *Machine Learning 24*(2), 123–140.

Breiman, L. (1998). Arcing Classifiers. *The Annals of Statistics 26*(3), 801–849.

Breiman, L. (2001). Random Forests. *Machine Learning 45*(1), 5–32.

Breiman, L., J. H. Friedman, R. A. Olshen, and C. J. Stone (1984). *Classification and Regression Trees*. New York: Chapman and Hall.

Breslow, N. E. (1972). Contribution to Cox (1972). *Journal of the Royal Statistical Society Series B 34*(2), 216–217.

Breslow, N. E. (1974). Covariance Analysis of Censored Survival Data. *Biometrics 30*, 89–99.

Buzas, J. S. (1998). Unbiased Scores in Proportional Hazards Regression with Covariate Measurement Error. *Journal of Statistical Planning and Inference 67*, 247–257.

Carroll, R. J., D. Ruppert, L. A. Stefanski, and C. M. Crainiceanu (2006). *Measurement Error in Nonlinear Models* (2nd ed.). Chapman and Hall, London.

Chu, C. S. J., K. Hornik, and C. M. Kuan (1995). MOSUM Tests for Parameter Constancy. *Biometrika 82*(3), 603–617.

Cox, D. R. (1972). Regression Models and Life-Tables (with discussion). *Journal of the Royal Statistical Society Series B 34*(2), 187–220.

Cox, D. R. (1975). Partial Likelihood. *Biometrika 62*, 269–276.

Fahrmeir, L., A. Hamerle, and G. Tutz (1996). *Multivariate statistische Verfahren.* de Gruyter Verlag.

Gimenez, P., H. Bolfarine, and E. A. Colosimo (1999). Estimation in Weibull Regression Model with Measurement Error. *Communications in Statistics – Theory and Methods 28*(2), 495–510.

Gorfine, M., L. Hsu, and R. L. Prentice (2004). Nonparametric Correction for Covariate Measurement Error in a Stratified Cox Model. *Biostatistics 5*(1), 75–87.

Hansen, B. E. (1992). Testing for Parameter Instability in Linear Models. *Journal of Policy Modeling 14*(4), 517–533.

Hjort, N. L. and A. Koning (2002). Tests for Constancy of Model Parameters Over Time. *Nonparametric Statistics 14*, 113–132.

Hothorn, T., K. Hornik, C. Strobl, and A. Zeileis (2010). party: A Laboratory for Recursive Partytioning. R package version 0.9-99991, http://cran.r-project.org/package=party.

Hothorn, T., K. Hornik, and A. Zeileis (2006). Unbiased Recursive Partitioning: A Conditional Inference Framework. *Journal of Computational and Graphical Statistics 15*(3), 651–674.

Hothorn, T., F. Leisch, and A. Zeileis (2010). modeltools: Tools and Classes for Statistical Models. R package version 0.2-17, http://cran.r-project.org/package=party.

Hu, C. and D. Y. Lin (2002). Cox Regression with Covariate Measurement Error. *Scandinavian Journal of Statistics 29*, 637–655.

Hu, P., A. Tsiatis, and M. Davidian (1998). Estimating the Parameters in the Cox Model When Covariate Variables Are Measured with Error. *Biometrics 54*, 1407–1419.

Huang, Y. and C. Y. Wang (2000). Cox Regression with Accurate Covariate Unascertainable: A Nonparametric Correction Approach. *Journal of the American Statistical Association 95*, 1209–1219.

Kalbfleisch, J. D. and R. L. Prentice (2002). *The Statistical Analysis of Failure Time Data* (2nd ed.). John Wiley and Sons, New York.

Kong, F. H. and M. Gu (1999). Consistent Estimation in Cox Proportional Hazards Model with Covariate Measurement Errors. *Statistica Sinica 9*, 953–969.

Kong, F. H., W. Huang, and X. Li (1998). Estimating Survival Curves Under Proportional Hazards Model with Covariate Measurement Errors. *Scandinavian Journal of Statistics 25*, 573–587.

Kopf, J., T. Augustin, and C. Strobl (2010). The Potential of Model-Based Recursive Partitioning in the Social Sciences - Revisiting Ockham's Razor. Technical Report Number 88, Department of Statistics, Ludwig Maximilian University of Munich, Germany.

Leisch, F. and E. Dimitriadou (2010). *mlbench: Machine Learning Benchmark Problems*. R package version 2.0-0, http://CRAN.R-project.org/package=mlbench.

Li, Y. and L. Ryan (2006). Inference on Survival Data with Covariate Measurement Error – An Imputation-based Approach. *Scandinavian Journal of Statistics 33*, 169–190.

Liu, K., R. A. Stone, S. Mazumdar, P. R. Houck, and C. F. R. III (2004). Covariate Measurement Error in the Cox model: A Simulation Study. *Communications in Statistics – Simulation and Computation 33*(4), 1077–1093.

Morgan, J. N. and J. A. Sonquist (1963). Problems in the Analysis of Survey Data, and a Proposal. *Journal of the American Statistical Association 58*, 415–434.

Nakamura, T. (1990). Corrected Score Functions for Errors-in-Variables Models: Methodology and Application to Generalized Linear Models. *Biometrika 77*, 127–137.

Nakamura, T. (1992). Proportional Hazards Model with Covariates Subject to Measurement Error. *Biometrics 48*, 829–838.

Nyblom, J. (1989). Testing for the Constancy of Parameters Over Time. *Journal of the American Statistical Association 84*, 223–230.

Peto, R. (1972). Contribution to Cox (1972). *Journal of the Royal Statistical Society Series B 34*(2), 205–207.

Ploberger, W. and W. Krämer (1992). The CUSUM Test With OLS Residuals. *Econometrica 60*(2), 271–285.

Potapov, S., W. Adler, and M. Schmid (2011). *survAUC: Estimators of Prediction Accuracy for Time-to-Event Data.* R package version 1.0-1, http://CRAN. R-project.org/package=survAUC.

Prentice, R. L. (1982). Covariate Measurement Errors and Parameter Estimation in a Failure Time Regression Model. *Biometrika 69*, 331–342.

Quinlan, J. R. (1986). Induction of Decision Trees. *Machine Learning 1*(1), 81–106.

R Development Core Team (2010). *R: A Language and Environment for Statistical Computing.* Vienna, Austria: R Foundation for Statistical Computing. ISBN 3-900051-07-0, http://www.R-project.org.

Schemper, M. and R. Henderson (2000). Predictive Accuracy and Explained Variation in Cox Regression. *Biometrics 56*(1), 249–255.

Schmid, M., T. Hielscher, T. Augustin, and O. Gefeller (2011). A Robust Alternative to the Schemper–Henderson Estimator of Prediction Error. *Biometrics 67*(2), 524–535.

Stefanski, L. A. (1989). Unbiased Estimation of a Nonlinear Function of a Normal Mean with Application to Measurement Error Models. *Communications in Statistics – Theory and Methods 18*(12), 4335–4358.

Strobl, C., J. Kopf, and A. Zeileis (2010). A New Method for Detecting Differential Item Functioning in the Rasch Model. Technical Report Number 92, Department of Statistics, Ludwig Maximilian University of Munich, Germany.

Strobl, C., J. Malley, and G. Tutz (2009). An Introduction to Recursive Partitioning: Rationale, Application and Characteristics of Classification and Regression Trees, Bagging and Random Forests. *Psychological Method 14*(4), 323–348.

Strobl, C., F. Wickelmaier, and A. Zeileis (2010). Accounting for Individual Differences in Bradley-Terry Models by Means of Recursive Partitioning. *Journal of Educational and Behavioural Statistics.* forthcoming.

Therneau, T. and T. Lumley (2009). *survival: Survival Analysis, Including Penalised Likelihood.* R package version 2.35-8, http://CRAN.R-project.org/package=survival – Original R port by Thomas Lumley.

Wang, C. Y., L. Hsu, Z. D. Feng, and R. L. Prentice (1997). Regression Calibration in Failure Time Regression. *Biometrics 53*, 131–145.

Wen, C.-C. (2009). Semiparametric Maximum likelihood estimation in cox proportional hazards model with covariate measurement errors. *Metrika 72*(2), 199–217.

Yi, G. Y. and J. F. Lawless (2007). A Corrected Likelihood Method for the Proportional Hazards Model with Covariates Subject to Measurement Error. *Journal of Statistical Planning and Inference 137*, 1816–1828.

Zeileis, A. (2005). A Unified Approach to Structural Change Tests Based on ML scores, *F* Statistics, and OLS Residuals. *Econometric Reviews 24*(4), 445–466.

Zeileis, A. (2006). Object-oriented Computation of Sandwich Estimators. *Journal of Statistical Software 16*(9), 1–16. http://www.jstatsoft.org/v16/i09/.

Zeileis, A. and K. Hornik (2007). Generalized M-Fluctuation Tests for Parameter Instability. *Statistica Neerlandica 61*(4), 488–508.

Zeileis, A., T. Hothorn, and K. Hornik (2008). Model-Based Recursive Partitioning. *Journal of Computational and Graphical Statistics 17*(2), 492–514.

Zeileis, A., T. Hothorn, and K. Hornik (2010). party with the mob: Model-based Recursive Partitioning in **R**. R package version 0.9-99991.

Zucker, D. and D. Spiegelman (2008). Corrected Score Estimation in the Proportional Hazards Model with Misclassified Discrete Covariates. *Statistics in Medicine 27*(11), 1911–1933.